PRAISE FOR *REBUILD*

In *Rebuild*, Dr. Rob Zembroski provides a unique motivational and evidence-based guide for a healthy and active life. By drawing on the latest research, as well as his own journey to rebuild himself after cancer, and over twenty years of working with his patients, Dr. Z provides a clear guide on how to design your own diet and exercise program that meets your specific situation and needs. No fads or extremes, just sound advice rooted in solid scientific research and real experience. He makes the research accessible and understandable. He shows you how to apply it with simple do-it-yourself tools. And he shows you how to keep it all in perspective so you can sustain your changes for a lifetime. If you are looking for a breakthrough that can work in the real world—your real world—this is a must-read.

Miriam E. Nelson, PhD, nutrition scientist and international best-selling author of the "StrongWomen" book series

Recent experience shows us that man was never meant to have this easy access to food, especially processed foods. The concepts and teachings of Dr. Z offer the reader insights into how to navigate modern-day food choices in a way that can clearly impact one's health and well-being.

Marc S. Penn, MD, PhD, FACC, Chief Medical Officer, Cleveland HeartLab, Inc.

A *terrific* book! The focus is on helping you create a *customized* nutritional and exercise regimen that's going to get *you,* in particular, out of the dangerous American swamp of idleness and lousy food. Rob is a solid, scientific thinker and an inspirational writer. He has made a difference in countless lives, and he will make a difference in yours.

Chris Crowley, best-selling co-author of the "Younger Next Year" books and **Thinner This Year**

Whether you are recovering from heart disease, cancer, or just trying not to *become* a statistic, *Rebuild with Dr. Z's Body Composition Diet* makes the mechanics of fat loss both possible and palatable. As upbeat and approachable as the doctor himself, it draws from the author's own battle with cancer, as well as case studies of success with his patients. Dr. Z's diet rules are sane, thoughtful guidelines within which you can wiggle: You can calculate the amount of food you should eat based on your metabolism, then create your *own* diet. Dr. Zembroski offers a truly comprehensive healing-and-weight-loss plan that is local-farm friendly and carefully supports the reader—from doing the body-composition math, to meal-plan prep and substitutions, and workouts. Bravo!

Belisa Vranich, PsyD, clinical psychologist and author of **Get a Grip: Your Two-Week Mental Makeover**

Over 50 percent of those having a heart attack or stroke had normal cholesterol levels, which proves it is essential to go beyond just lowering cholesterol. Adapting your lifestyle to Dr. Z's program will contribute to an overall healthy heart. Dr. Z's high-intensity interval training, along with his expert nutritional advice, can assist in preventing and reducing the buildup of calcification and plaque in your artery walls, which will lessen your overall chances of a cardiac event.

Jake Orville, President & CEO, Cleveland HeartLab, Inc.

REBUILD

WITH DR. Z's BODY COMPOSITION

D I E T

Dr. Robert Zembroski, DC, DACNB, MS

Two Harbors Press
322 First Avenue N, 5th floor
Minneapolis, MN 55401
612.455.2293
www.TwoHarborsPress.com

ISBN-13: 978-1-62652-775-1
LCCN: 2014904270

Distributed by Itasca Books

Front and back cover designs by Rui Weidt
Front-cover photograph by Christine Simmons
Back-cover "rebuilt" photograph by Ludwig Araujo

- All exercise graphics/illustrations ©Visual Health Information
- Interior photographs from iStock.com
©iStock.com/Yuri, ©iStock.com/cdwheatley, ©iStock.com/MarsBars, ©iStock.com/Shanekato, ©iStock.com/mujdatuzel, ©iStock.com/ YvanDube, ©iStock.com/michaelmjc, ©iStock.com/RobLopshire, ©iStock.com/BlueLemonPhoto, ©iStock.com/fcafotodigital, ©iStock. com/ivstiv, ©iStock.com/Scanrail, ©iStock.com/Ju-Lee, ©iStock. com/frender, ©iStock.com/minimal, ©iStock.com/mcfields, ©iStock. com/Imageegaml, ©iStock.com/pictafolio, ©iStock.com/jonnyscriv, ©iStock.com/AlexRaths, ©iStock.com/ugurhan, ©iStock.com/ CEFutcher, ©istock.com/TommL

Printed in the United States of America

To those with health challenges
who seek to go beyond survival and live free of disease.

To those looking for real answers
to losing fat without the frustrations of fad diets.

Acknowledgments

My very grateful appreciation to Christine "Misty" Barth, my office manager and dear friend, for helping me bring this book to life. Her impeccable editing skills and attention to detail are admirable. I can't thank Misty enough for her willingness to go the extra step and give her time so generously.

I thank my wife, Holly Bliss, for her loving and unwavering support over the last couple of years. Her coaching skills shine through, as evidenced in her contributions to the book.

Special thanks to Dr. Jeffrey Bland, whose inspiration and teachings have allowed me to rebuild myself, as well as encouraged me to help others do the same.

I thank freelance editor John Paine, who took my thoughts and research and created a cohesive storyline. I appreciate his guidance throughout the writing experience.

My appreciation to Rui Weidt for his outstanding creative work on the cover designs. On each of our projects, his talent continues to exceed my expectations.

Thanks to Dorian Barth and especially Yve Novotny for their delicious and nutritious recipes. I appreciate Yve's ability to infuse her recipes with creativity and enthusiasm.

My grateful thanks to Dave and Peg Bliss for their ideas, encouragement and support during the writing process.

Thanks also to Susan Kunin for her ideas, experience, and loyal support.

Last but certainly not least, my thanks to those patients who allowed the use of their personal stories.

Foreword

I have had the privilege of knowing Dr. Robert Zembroski for the past seven years, and I have found him to be an inspiration. His successful victory over cancer is only a part of his remarkable story. He is a person who "walks the talk." Through his advocacy he has helped his patients achieve amazing results with their health. So, this begs the question: "Why another diet book?" I have reviewed hundreds of diet books over the past thirty years in my career as medical researcher, educator, and opinion leader in nutrition and functional medicine. Most diet books are variations of the same theme: eat less, exercise more. There is some of that in Dr. Zembroski's book, *Rebuild*, but there is so much more to it. I found it compelling in the way he has woven his advocacy for health and vitality into the diet plan. I found that it reads less like a traditional diet book, rather more like a manifesto of the remarkable, and sometimes even miraculous, things that can happen when people take charge of their health.

I found the case histories from Dr. Z's practice to be compelling; they added life and reality to the message. The reader can feel the passion and pursuit of excellence that Dr. Z brings to his practice. You can also see that he is an accomplished professional in the exercise and nutrition sciences. His Master's degree in Science serves him well in the development of the well-grounded program that is described in the book.

As I read the book, I reflected on the conversations I have had with Dr. Z over the years and asked myself, "What makes certain people special?" My answer is that every person is special, but some have had life experiences that bring their "specialness" to a higher degree of visibility. Such is certainly the case with Dr. Z. He was a special breed of doctor before his experience with cancer, but after that experience his clarity of vision and commitment to helping others rose to new levels. This quality that makes Dr. Z special comes through loud and clear in the book. It motivates readers to want to do better, to take charge of their lives, and to commit to something that they may have thought was too hard before reading the book.

It is my belief that the biggest obstacle most people face when making meaningful changes in lifestyle and behavior is the inability to see beyond the sacrifice of the change to the payoff of improved health and vitality. This is where coaching and a positive support system come in. Dr. Z has written a book that provides reinforcement and step-by-step encouragement that pushes through the moments of doubt when we ask, "Is it worth it?" His story demonstrates that, "Yes, it is worth it," and it can happen to anyone following his program with commitment.

It has been a great pleasure to get to know Dr. Z over the years. It is the next step in my respect for him to see the results of his program of health and fitness now being translated for use by anyone reading his book. It is hard to know how many people are changed for the better by reading a book. I expect the number of success stories created by Dr. Z's program will be significant.

Jeffrey Bland, PhD, FACN, FACB
President and Founder
Personalized Lifestyle Medicine Institute
Seattle, Washington
www.plminstitute.org

CONTENTS

Introduction

Can you recover from heart disease, cancer, diabetes, obesity, or autoimmune issues, and actually be *healthier* than you were before you got sick? Let's say you found a plan that helped you lose toxic fat and increase your lean muscle, while preventing and reversing chronic disease at the same time. Would you stick to a plan like that?

In *Rebuild*, I explain how your body really loses weight, while improving your health. I present the latest research in an easy-to-read format, as well as the steps you need to create the body you want. Along the way you'll achieve the good health you deserve.

If you want proven scientific facts about the best ways to lose fat without starving yourself or wasting hours at the gym, this is the book for you. If you are looking for a guide to rebuild after an illness, restore your health, and prevent disease, this is the book for you. If you are looking for someone with personal experience to share honest information about the link between an unhealthful lifestyle and the creation of disease, this is the book for you. Using the information in *Rebuild*, you can create a lifestyle that will not only help you look great, you'll also have lots of energy and feel good about yourself.

My career is based on helping people resolve health issues by finding the root causes of their problems. Whether it's heart disease, cancer, hormone-based problems, chronic pain, fatigue, or weight issues, I take a functional approach to look for clues. I dig deep to understand the mechanisms of each issue in order to provide a way to reverse the cause and thus create health and normal function. I know that what I'm sharing with you works because it worked for me, and it has worked for countless patients.

Who am I? My name is Dr. Robert Zembroski, or "Dr. Z," as my patients call me. After a few short years of feeling intense stress and neglecting a healthful lifestyle, at 38 years old I was diagnosed with non-Hodgkin's lymphoma, a life-threatening blood cancer. The diagnosis took me by surprise. The first symptoms had been mild; I started losing muscle weight and developed a low-grade fatigue that no amount of caffeine and B vitamins would help. As the symptoms became more severe, along with intense head pain I was awakened by gushing night sweats. At that point I knew I was in trouble. I had blood work and x-rays done to find the reasons for my symptoms.

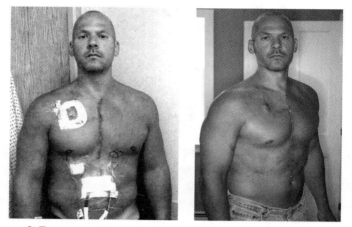

2 Days post-surgery   2 Months later

On August 18, 2006, a radiologist announced, "You have a five-inch tumor in your chest." The news caused the thoughts that had been scrambling around in my head to stop. My heart stopped beating, my blood stopped circulating, and voices sounded muffled. As I walked out of the doctor's office that day, I realized I had created my own disease by not taking care of myself.

Within a two-year period, I had seven months of the most toxic chemotherapy—including a chemical similar to mustard gas and a noxious substance called "red death"— and four weeks of radiation. Finally, a surgeon cracked open my chest from throat to belly and removed the mass of scar tissue where once a giant ball of cancer cells had been. The side effects of the toxic drugs and surgery left me weak and fatigued. Functional testing revealed a low red-blood-cell count, low platelets, and low white blood cells. My thyroid was affected, which created low thyroid hormones and the symptoms associated with hypothyroid (weak thyroid). These included fatigue, low energy, cold hands and feet, slow metabolism and dry skin. Hormone testing revealed low testosterone and low vitamin-D levels. The drugs also caused malabsorption of B vitamins as seen through a special test to check my metabolism and energy production. On top of discolored skin on my lower left leg from "red death," and collapsed veins in my arms, I suffered from residual tingling in my fingers, as well as weakness in the muscles of my lower left leg, which made fast walking or running a problem. Last, one of the chemo drugs affected my bladder, which delayed the sensation of urgency when I had to urinate. When I finally felt like I had to go…I *really* had to go.

Going forward, I knew I would need to learn what had caused my illness, as well as how to rehabilitate my body from the side effects of the cancer therapies. My goal was to prevent recurrence and create the ultimate healthy body—one that was disease-free, low-fat and lean. Reading through research on nutrition, nutritional biochemistry, genetics, cancer, endocrinology (the study of hormones), chronic disease, and exercise physiology, I developed a protocol for myself with one

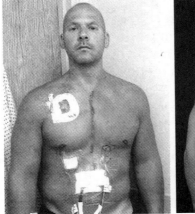 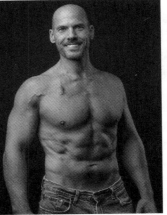

2 days post-surgery   5 years later

thing in mind—rebuild. Following this plan, I have improved my low blood counts, and restored my thyroid, testosterone and vitamin-D levels. My energy is back to normal, and the tingling in my limbs is gone. Frantically pulling off the next exit to empty my bladder is a problem of the past. Although the discolored skin remains, the weakness in my left leg is no longer interfering with my physical activity. Currently, I am lean with 10 percent body fat.

My personal experience, coupled with countless hours of research, has ignited in me a passion to help others resolve their health issues, so they don't have to go through what I experienced. Facing the grim reaper is not fun! Enduring debilitating and scarring procedures is not fun! As I continued to study the scientific research, I started to realize that the key to being healthy is also the key to being fit. I could not only prevent my cancer from coming back and rebuild myself from the destructive drugs and surgery; I could also change the composition of my body so that it would be lean.

We've all seen diet books touting some new fad plan. Others promote some gimmicky workout or fat-burning supplement. How many times have we seen a smiling celebrity on a book cover promising we'll "lose 21 pounds in 7 days"? Something grabs our attention, and off we go again. Three months later, we've regained all the pounds we lost—often more.

Most diets don't work because they are too extreme. Dieting is a lifestyle. The only permanent way to become slim, strong, and healthy is to make realistic changes. That means laying out realistic goals. Setting your sights only on the finish line can be overwhelming.

Instead, you can take small, incremental steps, similar to a runner looking for the next telephone pole while running a marathon. *Rebuild* helps you celebrate small wins while on your journey, an important way to move forward. Unless you focus on your progress, your old, unhealthful habits can sneak back in. When that happens, the fat comes back, and you stop exercising. Soon your health problem returns. Then you realize it's "another diet that didn't work."

Before I outline the Body Composition Diet for you, I'd like to the set the record straight by clarifying the definition of "diet." The word conjures up thoughts of short durations of restriction and starvation, where you have to give up foods you like for boring and tasteless "health food." You decide to go on a diet to get rid of fat, lose weight, or improve your health. The decision is less painful because the diet is for a short time; soon you can go off it and resume eating the way you did before. That mindset doesn't work because it creates only momentary famine. Then you indulge in rebound feasting on the processed and unhealthful foods that created your disease and altered body composition—one of being over-fat.

Somewhere along the line, the real meaning of diet has been misunderstood as a jail sentence of eating gruel. The word "diet" really refers just to the type of food you eat regularly, on a daily or weekly basis. Some people choose to eat only plant-based foods; others eat foods high in animal protein and low in carbohydrates. Many people eat anything and everything. Simply put, the foods you eat on a regular basis make up your diet.

Your body's composition consists of a mixture of elements that create a synergy of normal function and health. It also consists of different types of tissues, such as fat and muscle. To have a healthy body composition, you need an abundance of nutrients found in a variety of foods, as well as exercise to burn fat, tone muscles, and regulate the hormones that, in turn, control fat and muscle. Having a healthy body composition also depends on the alignment of additional factors, including stress management, elimination of environmental toxins, and a good night's sleep.

The Body Composition Diet goes far beyond getting rid of fat and losing weight. It is a research-based plan that you can use to rebuild after an illness, prevent disease, and restore the excellent health you deserve. The best thing about this approach is that you create a food plan that suits your metabolism and your specific health issues—like a custom suit or a ring that fits your finger just right. I will teach you how to do it by providing the do's and don'ts to create your custom program.

As I considered the negative mindset around the word diet, I wondered if I could somehow make the definition more appealing. I came up with an acronym for the word diet: Decide, Indulge, Enjoy and Transform. With that new focus, I broke it down into greater detail. When restoring your health, the first thing you have to do is **DECIDE**. As I say to my patients, the first step to resolving any health issue is *making a decision.* Once you make the decision, **INDULGE** in a variety of healthful foods that will force your body to burn fat and build lean muscle. Indulge in a variety of nutrient-dense and tasty whole foods that will communicate with your cells to turn on genes that create normal function, while at the same time shutting off genes that set the stage for disease. Doing that enables you to **ENJOY** the fruits of your effort with more energy, vibrancy and health. Enjoy looking better and leaner. Enjoy buying the clothes that help you look as good as you feel. Finally, watch yourself **TRANSFORM** physically and aesthetically. Transform yourself into the physically fit and healthy person you deserve to be.

You can find even more information by visiting my website at www.drzembroski.com. I look forward to hearing from you. I would also love to share your wins with others. You can inspire others to adopt new lifestyles for their own ultimate health and well-being!

I am excited to present a program based on scientific research that includes a simple outline for creating your own plan. Yes, you can rebuild after an illness, restore your health, prevent disease, and get rid of unwanted toxic body fat. The commitment and drive I had for myself, I now have for you.

What I did for myself, I can do for you.

DECIDE

I

E

T

Start Your New Day

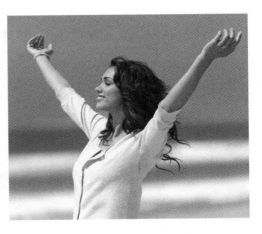

No more wishing for a better you. You're ready to take the reins and create the life and body you deserve. It's amazing to see the chain of positive events that can occur just by making a passionate, conscious decision to choose yourself over your excuses. Listen, we all get stuck. We find ourselves caught in the current of life floating downstream without an anchor. Yet drift isn't permanent, nor is it fate.

If we created it, we can change it. Your health destiny can be changed and *will be changed*. From time to time everyone needs a life raft, and you're looking at yours. Life is so much sweeter and abundant when we honor ourselves. It is time to change the outdated and self-defeating concept that we must persevere on our own with no assistance. The old way—"I'm tough, and I don't need anyone"—is a bunch of crap. We are social beings by nature, so reaching for support when we are trying to make real changes in life actually demonstrates strength and courage. *Rebuild* will, without a doubt, give you the tools and support you need to reach your goals.

I Lost 30 Pounds and Lowered My Cholesterol

A recent physical exam had uncovered high cholesterol, elevated blood pressure, and excess body fat. In addition, I was always tired and had little energy or stamina for anything other than work. At 51 years of age, I knew that it would become increasingly difficult for me to make and sustain the changes necessary to regain my health and energy. I needed to lose weight, eat better, and exercise. After several years of a sedentary lifestyle, I understood that changes were necessary, but was put off by my perception of how difficult they would be to make.

I can honestly say that one consultative meeting with Dr. Z is all it took to motivate me and get me moving forward. Why? Because his passion and enthusiasm are contagious, but, moreover, because he makes it simple.

The thing about most "diets" is that, by their very design, they are unsustainable for long periods of time and, therefore, temporary in nature. They can assist people in losing large amounts of weight relatively quickly, after which most eventually go back to their old ways. The difference in working with Dr. Z is that you move forward with changes in lifestyle that are gradual and easy to adopt.

I am happy to say that since I started working with Dr. Z, I have lost 30 pounds, cut my body-fat percentage in half, and lowered my cholesterol and blood pressure. I have more energy to do the things I enjoy outside of work.

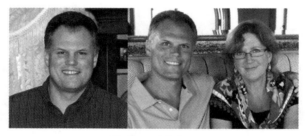

Before / After

I enthusiastically recommend Dr. Zembroski to anyone who wants to lose weight, gain energy, and get healthier. You will not find a stronger advocate for your health than Dr. Z . . . I guarantee it!

—Frank O.

Transform your mind. Frank was able to lose 30 pounds of body fat, as well as lower his blood pressure and cholesterol, because he made a decision. He chose not only to lose the fat, but also to get healthy by changing the way he ate and putting exercise back into his life. Making a decision to change your lifestyle is the first step to changing your body composition and restoring your health.

You say you've already made the decision to restore your health or lose weight, or you want to prevent disease. That's why you're reading this book. Great! You have taken the first step. Transformation begins with making a clear decision to change and having the positive mindset to carry you through the ups and downs in the journey. The second step is to find the tools, support, and guidance to turn your decision into a reality. The tools in this book are highly effective in helping you to reach your goals, if you apply them.

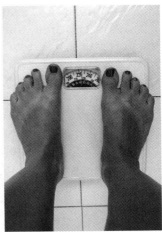

When patients first come to see me with their lists of health issues, I tell them the "cure" or solution to their ill health is to make a decision to get well and to do whatever it takes to get there. First, let's make sure about that decision. Find some uninterrupted "me time" to ask yourself, "Why am I doing this now?" "Am I ready to examine some of my old patterns so I can truly change?" "What is my mindset about getting healthy?" "What does 'healthy' even look like and feel like?" "What are the consequences if I don't change my ways?" This might be the first time you've needed to lose a few pounds, or maybe you're like so many others who have been "dieting" their entire lives. Perhaps you are now dealing with an unexpected health issue. That's why getting personal with yourself is so important.

Shana Y. says, "You gave me the tools; I have the discipline. It's encouraging and motivating to see change and progress so quickly. The foods I'm supposed to be eating are readily available and taste great! My goal now is to change the whole family."

The simple tools in this book are easy to incorporate into your life. However, in order for them to work, you need to find the inspiration—that emotional key that will create a permanent motivation for you to embody a long-term healthful lifestyle. Perhaps you want to continue to enjoy time with your children, family and friends, or you want to swing the golf clubs again, or get back to walking, biking, or skiing. Maybe you don't want to be the one who is chronically ill, taking lots of pills and unable to enjoy life. I was once asked why I kept the lights on in my practice. Not in a literal sense, but asking why I continue to do what I do—helping people get well, and coaching them along the way. Digging deeper into my emotions, I realized the reason I keep my lights on is to help people get well and to take away the fear and confusion, as well as that feeling of being overwhelmed, for those in search of answers to their health problems.

Any change in life takes commitment, consistency, support, tools, and a sense of humor. As Dr. Jeffrey Bland said, "The biggest obstacle most people face when making meaningful changes in lifestyle and behavior is the inability to see beyond the sacrifice of the change to the payoff of improved health and vitality."

It takes courage to say with conviction that you will be healthy, fit, and vibrant. It also takes a commitment to making the long-term changes necessary to resolve your health issues and get lean. However, what's the alternative? Popping pills forever? Getting disfiguring surgeries? Being disabled or lethargic and unable to enjoy life? Depending on your starting point, you may feel that you're kidding yourself because you can't even see your toes. You may be taking a bucket full of pills and wonder if it's even possible to stop taking them. Perhaps, like many others, you feel that the condition you have is just something you have to live with. Well, you don't. Telling yourself you can + believing it = results. My own story is a testament to how believing in yourself can alter your life.

I hope you can use it as an inspiration to change what you tell yourself about who you are.

Dr. Z's Confession

I sure didn't start in the place I am now. When I was a kid, I ate SpaghettiOs, Big Macs and Whoppers, grilled-cheese sandwiches, and peanut butter and fluff on white bread. I devoured Cap'n Crunch cereal and drank Kool-Aid every day. My siblings and I had access to this crap all the time; while we did eat a somewhat healthful dinner, that was really the only time we ate good food. Yep, I had "PFD"—what I've come to call Processed-Food Disorder. That high-calorie, low-nutrient, processed, refined junk made me chubby (OK, fat. Let's be honest, my nickname was Moose). I became addicted to junk food, which made me hyperactive. Moreover, I was prone to upper respiratory infections that seemed to last for weeks, coupled with seasonal allergies that no medication could touch. In fact, the antibiotics I took to fight the infections would create spotty rashes all over my body. My parents were, like most, too misinformed about nutrition to realize the serious effects a processed-food diet can have on the mind, body, and health. My hyperactivity got so bad that they actually bought books on how to cook for a hyperactive child! If you feed a normal, active boy a high-sugar, processed-food diet, then why are you scratching your head wondering why he seems so hard to handle?

I was fortunate to grow up in a great neighborhood with lots of kids of all ages. We played football, soccer, and baseball, and rode bikes everywhere for miles. We climbed trees, built forts, and explored the woods every chance we got. During the winter, we had snowball fights, built igloos, and played in the snow until our clothes were soaked. Every winter my older brothers and their friends created the ultimate high-speed sled-and-toboggan trail for the neighborhood by icing down an old horse trail. It was so much fun! At the opposite end of the year, when summer started, we thought of only one thing: endless days of fun in the sun with our friends, thrashing around in a swimming pool. Yet I was also filled with low self-esteem and embarrassment. I wore a T-shirt with my bathing suit because I was overweight and embarrassed to be seen with my shirt off. I wanted the T-shirt to hide my body; instead I had a wet, see-through T-shirt that stuck to me like flypaper. Somehow my enjoyment of the water kept me swimming despite the torment to my self-esteem.

In junior high school, as my height increased, my waistline decreased ever so slightly. I wore long pants and shirts that covered me up during these two years prior to high school. Then I realized I soon would be going to high school. That meant upperclassmen, girls, and sports. Feeling the pressures of a new environment and the dread of how others would perceive me, the race to lose the fat was on. I began exercising every day—running a mile or two every night, lifting cement-filled weights in the basement, and changing my diet to include nothing but vegetables and protein. I even drank vinegar because I heard it would help to melt the fat. Well, during that summer before high school, I lost most of the unwanted fat, saw muscle growth, and then felt comfortable enough to start high school, which is always a time when kids are so self-conscious. My allergies also improved, and sinus infections became an issue of the past.

I felt liberated from the chains of embarrassment over how I felt about myself and how I'd be perceived. You, too, can break your chains with the Body Composition Diet.

Changing into the New You

Of course, most adults do not exercise as much as teenagers, but we do have a lot more ability to change our circumstances. We can see what others are doing and say, "Hey, that's what I want" or "Whoa, I don't want to be like that."

Imagine how good it would feel to have someone say to you, "Wow, you look great!" Imagine getting up every day feeling energized, vibrant, and excited about life. Imagine seeing yourself lean, fit, feeling great, and full of energy. Think about how good it would feel knowing that you can control your health. How would it feel not to need medications and deal with the unending list of side effects? I bet you're smiling right now and have goose bumps. If so, you're giving yourself permission to believe, because you know you will achieve it. We've all had days of feeling insecure, not motivated, and not liking how we look or feel. Social events come up, and you want to get out there. Say you're meeting with friends you haven't seen in a while, and you start talking to yourself. "What will they say?" "Ugh, I put on weight and can't fit into my clothing." Or, you don't want to be intimate with your partner with the lights on because you don't like how you look. We all have had days of feeling terrible, when the worst part was getting through the workday or social gathering with a poker face while not showing your discomfort. During my cancer treatment, when seeing patients I can remember feeling ill and tired while my fingers tingled in pain and my eyes burned from the toxic side effects of chemotherapy. I couldn't wait until the nightmare was over and I could feel good again. I was already staring at the finish line.

Perhaps the worst part is the lack of control. When diagnosed with a health crisis, you may hear one thing from your doctor, but other advice from your friends and family about how to treat the condition. Or, like many, you stare at the computer reading through websites in hope of finding a solution. Both situations compound the worry and lack of control because you just want answers. You've gone through cancer treatment, had stents put into your arteries, or endured any one of a number of other procedures. Now you're looking for information and the tools to rebuild yourself and, of course, prevent recurrence. This lack of control can be overwhelming.

With poor eating habits, you may find yourself spinning out of control. Your waist size increases, and the next thing you know you're in the yo-yo dieting spiral, frustrated because you can't get rid of the fat. It's similar to the feeling of giving up control to a doctor who knows nothing about you—how you feel or what you're experiencing. You want to trust that he or she can help you figure out what's causing your ailment. You also don't want to feel like just another number. A lack of control creates frustration and negative emotions; eventually you give up because it's become too hard. Don't give up! If you give up on your body, it will give up on you.

If these thoughts have ever gone through your head, I can assure you that they will vanish once you start to rebuild. Instead, you'll enjoy the new you. First, you won't be part of the plus-size club anymore. That person no longer exists and isn't coming back. Shopping will be something you look forward to because you feel hot instead of frumpy. It feels amazing to have an entire store in which to shop instead of just one section. We may fool ourselves into thinking otherwise when we are over-fat, but deep down, you know it doesn't feel good to shop in a section that labels you as beyond standard sizing. Second, you will have lots of energy and improved health to enjoy the things you love to do.

This diet does not call for starvation, restriction, punishment, or guilt if you fall off the wagon. I'm not asking you to make false promises and set unrealistic goals. Your perception of dieting—changing what you eat, letting go of old habits, replacing your comfort foods, etc.—may make change seem too difficult and restrictive. That's why the majority of weight-loss diets consist of quick fixes and gimmicks designed to get you pumped up for change. The problem is they leave you discouraged, depleted, and usually heavier than when you started. Not this one—not this time! The key to losing fat, gaining 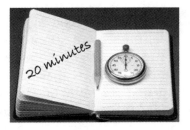 lean muscle and restoring your health is *not* a mystery. It is not difficult, nor does it have to be boring.

So if you are about to say, "I can't," immediately correct yourself and say, "I can." Usually, "I can't" really means "I'm scared/confused/frustrated" or "I don't know where to begin." Whatever has prevented you from taking action, acknowledge it and let it go. "Can't" is no longer a part of your inner dialogue. What you tell yourself with conviction you can turn into reality. I have been there. Once I changed my thoughts, I changed my ways.

If you want some inspiration, think of how much more energy you'll have to do the things you love to do. As a society, we tend to shock ourselves awake and sedate ourselves to sleep! Imagine waking up full of energy and having enough to get you though the day. Getting rid of the fat will reduce your weight. The lighter you are, the less energy you will expend just to get around. If you carried a 50-pound backpack, you would quickly become exhausted, as well as cause damage to your joints. The same thing is true when you lose weight. Furthermore, by eliminating high-calorie foods, you will have fewer spikes in blood sugar and won't experience "sugar crashes" after each meal. By eating lean protein, healthful fat, high-fiber carbs, and nutrient-rich fruits, you will get the right amount of calories to provide constant energy all day.

A healthy body composition is about being low-fat and lean, not light and undernourished. Being light isn't the same as being healthy. Examples: a 45-year-old woman weighing 130 pounds with 35 percent body fat, or a 45-year-old man weighing 170 with a 28 percent body fat. For both, the body fat is too high. But the goal is not to lose the weight; it's to lose the fat. Many people who lose weight under other diet programs are actually losing muscle while retaining the fat. The scale shows a reduction in weight, but that person is still over-fat. Lean muscle is the fountain of youth. The more lean muscle you have, the more metabolically active you are. That state will allow you to burn fat and keep it off. The tips and tools in this book will allow you to do just that—lose the fat and save the muscle, at any age.

I should note that lots of diet books feature super-muscular men and women on the covers, giving you the impression that you can look like that. (By the way, you can.) However, the information in those books is often unrealistic when someone actually tries to achieve that body type. Pictures of super-fit people can be inspiring but also very daunting. The problem is, up until now you just haven't had the right tools and support to match your inner desire to change. Getting lean and healthy is accomplished by working smarter, not harder.

What does that really mean? How about less time working out? Long periods of endurance exercise have long been associated with burning fat. Gyms are filled with people running, oscillating, and climbing stairs for hours on end in the hope of melting body fat. Yet most people find that long-term exercise with moderate intensity does not produce the fat loss they expected. Research—as well as my own personal experience—shows that high-intensity exercise for short periods is the best way to burn fat. High-intensity interval training (HIIT) typically involves all-out intensity for a short period, followed by periods of low-intensity exercise or rest. A great example of this is sprinting—explosive movement for a short time, followed by a walk or rest.

"I don't have time to spend an hour or more at the gym." This is what I hear all the time from patients who are trying to lose weight and improve their health. In fact, many people give up because they get frustrated thinking they have to exercise all day to get in shape or recover from a health crisis. Over-training can cause injury and an inability to lose fat. So get ready for this announcement: You can get rid of the fat, get lean, and turn your health around in a fraction of the time you once dreaded. High-intensity training takes only 20 minutes to get you lean and healthy.

I can hear the doubts now. Promises, promises . . . 20 minutes, good health . . . That's because lots of diet/health books have their special twist, their hook. *Rebuild* isn't like that. It is based on the latest scientific research. This plan has no gimmicks or quick fixes—just proven, easy-to-follow steps that will take you from a decision for change to real results. As you shed the fat and gain lean muscle, you will also be reversing chronic illness, increasing longevity, and gaining abundant energy to do all the things you love. If that doesn't get you excited, you need to figure out what's holding you back. We all want to be healthy, happy, and abundant in our lives.

That's the true advantage of this program. Losing fat, feeling great, and looking amazing are, of course, the obvious perks, but the real gift lies in the major health benefits of reversing and preventing disease. I don't know about you, but if I knew that changing my body composition would prevent me—or my loved ones—from getting cancer, diabetes, Alzheimer's disease, and heart disease, I would be all over making these simple changes in order to have a life that is disease free. Trust me, a fast-food burger, deep-fried foods, chips, bottles of soda, or any of the other processed foods we consume are not worth having to fight for your life. Many times I hear patients say, "I'll die if I can't have my ice cream, soda . . . I can't live without it!" My answer is, "You may not live with it."

News flash! "Hurricane Whopper is set to hit land today, bringing heavy rain and strong winds which can damage buildings, cars, and trees. The storm surge will create big waves which can erode beaches and destroy homes on the water." When we eat processed foods, we are like that accident waiting to happen. Although you know the hurricane is coming, you wait until the day of the storm to buy batteries and water. Likewise, you know the oil in your car needs to be changed every 2,500 to 3,000 miles, but you wait until you've driven 5,000 miles. Last-minute holiday shopping is a nightmare, fighting the crowds and rummaging through the depleted merchandise to find that special gift. Why do we do that? Sadly, we do the same with our health. We skate along without thought or worry about health until . . . Bam! We have a heart attack or are diagnosed with cancer.

Unfortunately, we often don't make a change until we receive a serious diagnosis. Don't gamble any longer with your health! Be proactive. We all think disaster will never happen, but when it does, we wish we had done things differently. There is nothing fun about lying in a hospital bed, getting poked, cut open, infused with toxic chemicals and medication which make you feel sick and drained while life passes you by.

Experiences like mine are becoming more and more frequent these days. The *2008 Almanac of Chronic Diseases* reported that chronic diseases are a significant problem in the United States. "More than 133 million Americans, or 45 percent of the population, have at least one chronic condition. These include arthritis, asthma, cancer, cardiovascular (heart) disease, depression, and diabetes. Many chronic diseases are caused or exacerbated by poor nutrition, lack of exercise, smoking, and other lifestyle choices."

The research is clear on this point. The way we eat is responsible for creating most chronic diseases. In this country, coronary-artery disease affects nearly 17 million people. According to the *New England Journal of Medicine,* approximately half of people who suffer from a heart attack or stroke have normal cholesterol levels. Yet we are brainwashed to think we are "healthy" when we have normal cholesterol levels. If half of the people who suffer from heart attacks or strokes have normal cholesterol levels, why bother to test it? Did you know that, for many people, the first sign of a heart attack is death?

Clinical Note

Cholesterol has long been blamed for the development of atherosclerosis and coronary-artery disease. However, the theory that cholesterol sticks to and clogs arteries has been disproven. Atherosclerosis is an inflammatory condition that occurs in the wall of an artery. When this process becomes advanced, certain biochemicals leak out of the arteries into the blood, which indicate the extent of arterial damage. These biochemicals now can be tested to determine your risk for a heart attack, as well as the level of inflammation from initial stages to advanced disease. Current standards of care to determine your risk of heart disease are testing cholesterol, LDL, HDL, and triglycerides—all of which are liver-function tests, not tests for heart disease. For more information about this new, advanced testing, visit my website at www.drzembroski.com or www.darienfm.com. You can also send your questions regarding this testing to info@darienfm.com.

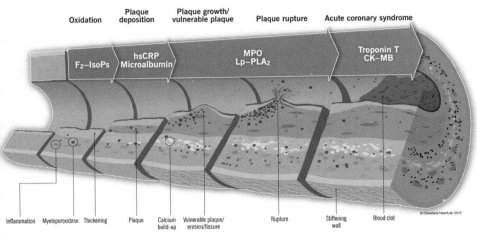

Oxidation	Plaque deposition	Plaque growth/ vulnerable plaque	Plaque rupture	Acute coronary syndrome

F_2–IsoPs | hsCRP Microalbumin | MPO Lp–PLA$_2$ | Troponin T CK–MB

Inflammation Myeloperoxidase Thickening   Plaque   Calcium build-up   Vulnerable plaque/ erosion/fissure   Rupture   Stiffening wall   Blood clot

© Cleveland HeartLab 2010

©Cleveland HeartLab.

The true culprit behind heart attack and stroke is inflammation. Not like the inflammation of a sprained ankle, but a swelling inside an artery, which causes a narrowing of the artery and reduced blood flow to the heart. The picture above does *not* show cholesterol clogging the artery. Instead, it illustrates inflammation in the wall of the artery. Inflammation is caused by a diet consisting of bad foods—in other words, an inflammatory diet.

For those of you who want more information on a topic, I have included details in the form of "Z Notes" placed throughout the book to provide additional science and/or further research. You can also choose to skip over those sections and continue reading.

Z Note

What is inflammation? Under normal circumstances, the inflammatory response, created by the immune system, is needed to fight foreign invaders and heal injuries. We can feel and see inflammation when there is pain, redness, and heat—a sore throat, a cut, a sprained ankle, and even a sunburn. Inflammation is a sign that the immune system is actively fighting infection and/or mending cells and tissues. This type of immune response should be short-lived. However, the body runs into trouble when the immune system runs out of control, creating chronic inflammation. Unmanaged, this type of inflammation can result in cancer, atherosclerosis and coronary-artery disease, autoimmune disease, and obesity. The extent of chronic inflammation is influenced by diet, physical inactivity, exposure to toxins, too much stress, and genetics.

Most chronic inflammation is caused by a diet consisting of processed food—otherwise known as an inflammatory diet. The good news is that a diet of high-nutrient, low-calorie foods contains all the right ingredients to prevent chronic inflammation in the arteries, thus lowering your risk for a heart attack or stroke. These foods include monounsaturated fats (cold-pressed olive oil), raw nuts, and seeds. Your allies are rainbow-colored and dark leafy vegetables, as well as low-sugar fruits like blueberries, blackberries, and strawberries. These food sources are loaded with antioxidants, which prevent inflammation in the arteries. In the next chapter, you will find more information about disease-fighting foods.

You can also help your cause by doing the right type of exercise. It's a well-known fact that high-intensity training and exercising prevents heart disease by reducing blood pressure, raising HDL, helping the body to use insulin to regulate blood sugar, moderating stress, and lowering body fat. Exercising, along with an anti-inflammatory diet, is the best medicine to prevent heart disease.

In 1971, President Richard Nixon declared war on cancer. Yet in the 40 years since, very little change has occurred in the cancer rate. That's not because we magically have inherited a new cancer gene. According to the World Cancer Research

Fund/American Institute for Cancer Research, the majority of cancers are not inherited. Only 5 to 10 percent of cancers are linked to single, inherited genes. *Pharmaceutical Research* published an article titled "Cancer Is a Preventable Disease That Requires Major Lifestyle Changes." The article starts by saying that scientists believe that the majority of cancer cases are preventable. The research goes on to say that 90 to 95 percent of all cases are rooted in the environment and lifestyle. In other words, if you are eating a processed, fast-food diet, are sedentary, or are inhaling and drinking toxins, you are creating an environment for the growth of cancer.

The development of cancer (carcinogenesis) is a multistep process caused by genetic errors that control normal cell function. These errors are actually mutations passed down to daughter cells, which may also develop additional mutations. An accumulation of these mutated cells is called a tumor. However, cancer develops only when these mutated cells have a survival advantage over normal neighboring cells.

Under normal circumstances, the ability of a cell to repair itself, thus preventing genetic errors, depends on nutrition and the appropriate intake of macronutrients—protein, fat, and carbs—and micronutrients—vitamins, minerals, and other compounds found in fruits and vegetables. If cancer does develop, the survival of those cancer cells depends also on the internal landscape of the body and the factors that promote cancer-cell survival and progression into a tumor. Fascinating research found in the *New England Journal of Medicine* states that only .01% of cancer cells that break off from a tumor (metastasis) survive inside the body. Their survival is dependent on the body's microenvironment. If the internal environment of the body is oxygen-rich and contains the appropriate nutrients, cancer cells won't survive.

All cells of the body have the ability to commit suicide when they are damaged or have become too old. This process of programmed cell death is called apoptosis. However, when this programmed cell death fails to happen, the immortalized cells can do more harm than good. This is a common scenario seen in cancer and tumor development. Mutated cells, as well as cells growing out of control, have turned off this suicide program, allowing them to survive in the body—this is cancer. *Pharmaceutical Research* also states that compounds found in foods like grapes and berries regulate this suicide program allowing cancer cells to die, as they should.

The fuel for cancer growth is a processed, nutrient-deprived diet, one that consists of junk sugar, artificial sweeteners, additives, partially hydrogenated vegetable oil, refined grains, sugar, and dairy—the typical Western diet. One spark for the growth of cancer is a hormone that most of us think is responsible for diabetes: insulin. While poorly managed blood sugar and insulin is the dysfunction behind diabetes, it—insulin—also contributes to the development of malignant colon cancer—the second most common cause of cancer morbidity (death) among men and women. Studies found in *The Journal of Nutrition* and *Cancer Causes and Control*, found high insulin (hyperinsulinemia) caused cells of the colon to mutate and grow. They also found visceral fat and obesity, physical inactivity, low levels of fiber and polyunsaturated fat to contribute to abnormal insulin levels and, thus, increase the risk for colon cancer.

As long as we're on the topic of diabetes, it should be stressed that type 2 diabetes is a chronic metabolic condition where cells resist or ignore insulin, resulting in high sugar levels in the blood. It is caused mainly by the way we eat. A number of research studies have found that years of eating lots of refined carbohydrates and processed foods with empty calories will flood your blood with sugar, causing a resulting flood of insulin. A diet of high sugar and refined carbs causes the cells to reject insulin. When cells reject insulin, sugar can't get into the cells, and hypoglycemia (low blood sugar) develops, increasing hunger and cravings for the same junk that created the problem. So you eat more, thus perpetuating the cycle.

The American Journal of Clinical Nutrition states that 16 million Americans have type 2 diabetes, and that one-third of them do not even know it. Recent data also suggests that 47 million

Americans have a condition called metabolic syndrome, an insulin resistance associated with type 2 diabetes. The main reason for this condition is an unhealthful lifestyle, which includes being overweight, sedentary, and, of course, eating a diet of refined carbohydrates, including refined grains and sugars. The complications from type 2 diabetes can include renal failure, erectile dysfunction, sleep apnea, blindness, slow-healing wounds (including surgical incisions), arterial disease, and coronary-artery disease.

To add salt to the wound, Alzheimer's disease, a neurodegenerative condition of the brain, is characterized by beta-amyloid deposits (plaques) in regions of the brain, resulting in cognitive decline and, eventually, death. Chronic diseases, including cancer, heart disease, type 2 diabetes, and Alzheimer's disease, are commonly blamed on inheritance and genetics. The scientific community, not the pharmaceutical community, says the opposite. According to the *Journal of Alzheimer's Disease*, genetic factors can predispose individuals to develop these plaques, but most cases of Alzheimer's disease-type dementia are sporadic and do not have a clear genetic link. What they found was most interesting.

The predominant reason behind the cause of Alzheimer's disease is improper insulin control, just as in type 2 diabetes. In fact, many researchers are calling Alzheimer's disease "type 3 diabetes." The results of the study suggest that the improper insulin signaling seen in Alzheimer's disease is also linked to free-radical damage (defined on page 69 in the vitamin and mineral section of the "Indulge" chapter) to brain cells, thus contributing to the formation of the plaques. With further investigating, the mechanism behind the development of type 2 diabetes is similar to the disease process that creates Alzheimer's disease.

The good news is that by getting rid of high-sugar, processed foods, and incorporating high-intensity exercise, you can improve your blood sugar and regulate your insulin. That means you can also decrease your chances of developing cancer, diabetes, metabolic syndrome, and Alzheimer's disease.

Rapid Weight Loss: Another Diet Trap?

Most fad or extreme diets promise rapid weight loss overnight. From counting points to severe calorie restriction coupled with hormone shots all the way to gastric-bypass surgery—these diets or procedures promise rapid weight loss. Don't like the idea of using surgery to tie up your stomach? Now there is an alternative. You can swallow stuff that fills your stomach so you are "forced" to eat less. To get you to buy into this, advertising for this procedure states that you still will be able to eat hot dogs, ice cream, cake, and pie, and you can forget about strict menus or calories because you are forced to eat less. However, you are still eating the foods that spike your fat-storing hormones, thus shutting down the fat-burning hormones. In the "Enjoy" chapter, I discuss those hormones in detail so you can learn how to master them.

Many times you have heard people claiming to lose lots of weight in a short period of time. Is there any factual basis to these claims, and can it be done? The key to quick weight loss is water. There is a principle in nutritional biochemistry that states, "Where sugar goes, water goes"; simply put, eating sugar causes water retention. "Miraculous" weight loss occurs when you stop eating processed sugars and carbs. Rapid, and oftentimes dramatic, loss of body weight is created by diet-induced diuresis (die-yur-resis), which is water loss when dieting. I'm sure you've heard of diuretics, or water pills, prescribed to people with high blood pressure. Diuretics work by making your kidneys dump sodium into the urine; this sodium takes water with it. The loss of water leads to a loss of blood volume and, subsequently, a loss in blood pressure.

In diets where carbohydrate intake is reduced, a couple of metabolic reactions occur. Before I describe these reactions, I think it's important to revisit sugar, especially its stored form, glycogen. When we eat carbohydrates, they are broken down into glucose and stored as glycogen in the liver and skeletal muscles. Glycogen acts as long-term energy storage along with the fat found in adipose tissue, which is the primary long-term energy source. For most people, dieting starts with cutting carbs, which then forces the body to use the stored glycogen as fuel. Here's where the water comes in: for every gram of glycogen stored in the liver and muscles, there are three grams of water stored with it.

Restricting carbs leads to the loss of glycogen. When this glycogen is lost, water is lost along with it. The more glycogen lost, the more water lost. Water is heavy; one gallon weighs eight pounds. So the promise of losing crazy amounts of weight in a short period of time does have some merit. However, this initial weight lost is not fat.

The second metabolic reaction that contributes to rapid weight loss also involves the elimination of water. When carbs are cut from the diet, the body begins breaking down fat. When that happens, biochemicals called ketone bodies are produced. When the fat cells deflate and release their fatty acids into the blood, those fatty acids end up in the liver and are broken down for energy, aka ketone bodies. The ketones are not only used for fuel, they also end up being filtered out by the kidneys, which, in turn, causes a loss of sodium and water.

I understand the desire to get rid of the fat quickly. However, not having the right tools or information about weight loss, fat loss, and body composition will ultimately lead to another diet that didn't work. Once you have the tools, you can be in complete control of your body composition and, most important, your health.

Are You Ready?

Let's get one thing straight. Being slim and healthy doesn't mean you have to stop eating everything you enjoy. This plan does not confine you to a jailhouse. You'll be able to enjoy lots of tasty food. While sitting with my patient Barb three weeks after she started her new diet, she expressed with excitement: "I no longer have to count points, and my sugar cravings went away after two weeks. I never thought I could go cold turkey from eating the sugary foods, but it was easy. I thought I could never live without breads, dairy, or sugar, but now it's easy. I've lost 10 pounds in three weeks!"

Foods that contain lots of salt, sugar, and fat can be addicting. Just like drugs, foods can excite certain parts of the brain, which cause you to crave more of the same junk. Food addictions, as well as using foods to self-medicate, also can cause you to get fat. As you eliminate high-calorie, processed foods, the cravings for these foods disappear. I promise! Once you get over the "craving" hump, your palate will change. Healthful food doesn't have to be boring. Who would have thought a salad filled with rainbow-colored vegetables and low-calorie, no-sugar dressing could taste so good? Savoring a bowl of steel-cut oats, topped with dark-red strawberries, sweet blueberries, and some crunchy walnuts, is a great way to start the day.

At the end of this book you will find delicious recipes to excite your taste buds, restore your health, and help you fight the battle of the bulge. Craving healthful foods will become a whole different type of addiction.

Here are some tips and tools that will help you throughout this amazing journey.

1. **Superhero.** Set your intention on creating a healthy, vibrant life for yourself. Everyone is different; you need to find what works for you. I grew up loving the comics, and the Hulk was my favorite character—super-strong and indestructible. My fascination with comic-book heroes was focused not only on good guy vs. bad guy; I was intrigued by the physiques they had and the way the artists drew them. I imagined myself muscular and strong like a superhero. Later in life, I found myself interested in how the body works. I pursued a career that would allow me to help people resolve their health issues, prevent disease, and get back into shape.

   Today, I still collect comic books, but instead of wanting to emulate superheroes, I use pictures of how I rebuilt myself after the cancer treatment—mustard gas, radiation, and surgery to remove the five-inch tumor from my chest. These photos keep me motivated to live a healthful lifestyle, and they remind me of what happens when you stop taking care of yourself.

   Now I have 10 percent body fat and incredible energy, and I am probably the healthiest I have ever been. My pictures remind me that no matter where you start from, or what obstacles you may see in front of you, there is nothing you can't do when you believe and commit. You may not aspire to reach the level of fitness I have, but the possibility is there. You have the opportunity to create the body you want. So, find your inspiration—a word or phrase, a picture of you at an ideal weight, the cover of a book, or a combination of inspirational ideas. Whatever it is, be committed to it every day. Being a healthy, vibrant person is not for a select few. Anyone who wants it and believes it can achieve it.

2. **Cheerleader.** Tell your partner, best friend, parent, or sibling about your goal and your commitment to change. Choose someone you know you can trust, who will be supportive and might even join you. This is very important! People close to you may feel threatened by

your change. There is a reason for the old saying "Misery loves company." Seeing someone close making positive changes often forces people to acknowledge what isn't working in their own lives. So, find a buddy who will truly support you. Maybe you will be lucky enough to get several people involved. If so, perhaps have everyone contribute a small amount to a kitty you can use to celebrate with a fun activity at the end of your first 30 days.

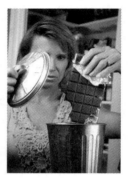

3. **Clean Start.** Put on some good music, grab a garbage bag, and get to work. Go through your refrigerator, pantry, and even your secret hiding places to start the process of letting go of all the processed foods, frozen dinners, cookies, chips, sodas—everything that no longer serves you. You'll find many food sources to replace your old addictions. Don't panic, fearing you will be eating only celery and carrot sticks. Trust me, this diet won't be restrictive and boring. When you're shopping for food, plan ahead. Think about preparing your meals and snacks, and try not to go food shopping when you are really hungry. Hunger sometimes plays tricks on our minds, causing us to gravitate toward processed foods.

4. **Outfitting.** Get yourself some new sneakers, a water bottle, and some comfortable workout clothes. This is an important investment in your commitment to a healthy you.

5. **Goals and Rewards.** You have your long-term goal, but you also must set up some short-term goals and rewards. Take the time to do something for yourself at the end of each week, or when you reach a short-term goal. This reward will be different for everyone, but here are some suggestions: new music for your iPod, a manicure, time at the driving range, a new book, or a

new outfit. Whatever it is, reward yourself for staying the course.

6. **Keeping Track.** Journaling is a great way to mark your journey, but I know this may not appeal to everyone. Making a spreadsheet or chart to post on the fridge is a good alternative. Do whatever works for you. I have also created the *Rebuild Logbook* to help you keep track of the foods you eat and the exercises you do. Keeping the Logbook in your purse or briefcase will allow quick and easy access to keep you going.

7. **Who Is That?** Take a picture when you start, because I guarantee you won't be the same person as you make progress. Many patients regret not taking a "before" picture to remind themselves of where they started. You never know; you may be chosen as a testimonial in the next book.

8. **Low Points.** Know your weak times during the day: when you have cravings, or when you feel overwhelmed, stressed, or fatigued. Have things in place to prevent you from going back to old habits like swinging by to grab some fast food or reaching for the TV remote and a bag of chips or cookies. If you have a smartphone, program it to pop up a positive reminder during your low points. When you feel hungry, drink water with a squeeze of lemon, or a cup of herbal tea, to satisfy your hunger. Other suggestions: Call a friend to distract you, take your dog for a walk . . . whatever works for you. This will keep you motivated. However, if you do slip back, don't beat yourself up. Just acknowledge it, brush yourself off, and move forward with a smile.

9. **Pay Attention.** Get to know your inner dialogue, your story, and your self-sabotaging ways. More often than not, you are usually your own biggest obstacle to reaching your goals. This is so important. When you start to tune in to your inner dialogue, you may be surprised at how often you say negative things about yourself. As soon as that happens, just redirect it to something

positive: "I can rebuild myself." "I can be healthy and lean." It's OK if you don't fully believe your mantra yet. If you stay with it, you will change your inner dialogue and transform your ways. Pay attention also to the story about yourself that you share with others. Why are you being negative when you're doing something that is so positive?

10. **Rebuild.** Remember the ultimate goal is to get rid of body fat, prevent illness, and rebuild your health. I can remember sitting in the chemo room, thinking how much easier it would have been if I had resolved my stress and eaten the right healing foods. From that experience, I knew I would create a plan, a program to improve my health and rebuild from the toxic therapies. There is no greater asset than your health.

Getting a healthy body composition doesn't have to be bleak or frustrating. Actually, as you will see in later chapters, creating a lean and healthy body is the complete opposite of living a boring, restrictive lifestyle. Most diet books set you up to fail. That's kind of crazy, but totally true. What differentiates this book from the rest is incorporating the right tools at the right time. *Rebuild* is about enjoying, indulging, and transforming your life. You don't have to work harder; you have to work smarter. I promise: if you follow the steps in each chapter, you will break the cycle of yo-yo dieting and live the life you've always wanted.

Tom M. says, "I have made a difference in my life, which has affected people around me. I feel like a poster boy for Dr. Z. I am always asked, 'Tom, how did you lose all that weight? You look great!' My answer is simple: 'It's a lifestyle change.' I have referred many people to Dr. Z, and I continue to spread the word about how to live a longer life, with a healthier lifestyle." It's time to rebuild!

D

INDULGE

E

T

Why Most Diets Don't Work

Dieting has the reputation of being restrictive and boring—and ineffective, if you don't follow the diet rules. The "starve-yourself" mindset is entrenched in our culture. This paradigm of food restriction has led to the creation of hundreds of diet plans, each one with some new twist on the right way to lose weight.

The traditional dieting model promotes calorie restriction and endless hours on a treadmill. Just as medications treat symptoms of disease, traditional dieting treats the symptoms of being over-fat. It does not address the behaviors that cause excessive calorie consumption and a sedentary lifestyle. As a society, we are focused on getting rid of fat as fast as possible. For many this method doesn't work at all, or works only for the short term.

Listen, I get it. Changing your lifestyle can be hard. It requires changing your current habits. But that is the way to transform yourself: to create new habits that are more healthful in the long run. Change is hard only if you make it hard. Here is a quote from Lauren D.:

"Hi, Dr. Z. I wanted to give you an update since we met. I have lost five pounds, and I feel great! I never realized how easy it would be to give up cow pus (milk). I don't even miss it. I have almond milk in my coffee, and I don't even miss cheese. I am never hungry and, most important, I am not bloated. Wow! I don't even miss the pasta and bread. Just wanted to thank you so much, and I will definitely keep you posted."

Lauren used some of the simple steps in *Rebuild*, and she states it was easy. Losing the fat and getting lean requires some rethinking of ways of eating that you take for granted, but the process is not difficult once you have the right tools.

Starvation diets and major calorie restriction create changes in your body's metabolism that make getting rid of fat difficult. According to *Psychosomatic Medicine*, in an article titled "Low-Calorie Dieting Increases Cortisol," researchers found that major calorie restriction created elevated levels of cortisol (a hormone related to stress). Those elevated cortisol levels were caused by the mental stress of dieting. Yet the stress was also caused by a lack of energy (calories) from food. That's right, major calorie restriction causes the release of cortisol. 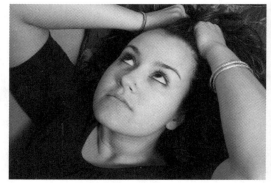 What does that hormone do? It breaks down muscle and turns it into sugar for the brain, while at the same time preserving body fat. Therefore, what all those diets say is wrong. Those diets turn on the wrong hormone. That's why severe food restriction can make you over-fat.

Living a healthful lifestyle that can be sustained over the long run is really the key for permanent fat loss. A lifestyle change will work if you set realistic goals, reward yourself along the way, and create a plan that is specific to you, one that you can stick to. Losing fat, maintaining muscle, and restoring health is a process, not a seven-day event. The place to start is looking at the food choices you make every day.

The Body Composition Diet works with your body. Certain foods turn on certain hormones that draw energy either from fat or from your muscles. You want to eat the foods that give your body the right signals. Once you understand how this process works, you, not some diet book, will be in charge.

I Lost 40 Pounds and Reduced My Risk for Heart Disease

Despite successful treatment for breast cancer, I was struggling with health issues: excess weight, joint problems, and unfavorable blood tests.

Dr. Z took time to review my entire medical history, including recent treatment for breast cancer. My blood tests showed elevated cholesterol, and he expressed concern about my risks for heart disease and other chronic illness.

Following his nutritional advice, I lost 40 pounds, cut my body fat from 36 percent to 29 percent, and my cholesterol level fell from 220 to 170. Best of all, I'm confident that I can maintain these health benefits due to a complete turnaround in my thinking about food and nutrition as "information" for my body's genes.

I posted my blood tests on my refrigerator door. So whenever I start to miss cheese and other former addictions, I look at my blood results and vow never to go back to my old ways.

At age 61, I have the energy to train for a local cancer charity bike ride.

Thanks, Z!

Mimi G.

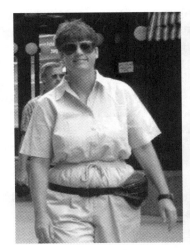 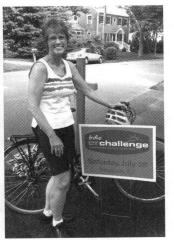

Before / After

Food Is the Control

What is food? What you eat provides you with much more than just fuel and energy. It provides you with the fundamental ingredients to make healthy bones, muscles, and skin. Food also provides the raw material to manufacture hormones and neurotransmitters, the biochemicals that allow you to think and feel.

All food—from burgers to a mixed-greens salad—is composed of three parts: macronutrients, micronutrients, and water. Let's look first at what macronutrients do. Food is made primarily of macronutrients, which can be broken into three more categories that everyone is familiar with: protein, fat, and carbohydrates. These food components provide energy, measured as calories, to maintain life. Without them we would suffer from malnutrition, starvation, and death. They play a second important role as well. Macronutrients help to regulate both the hormones that make us fat as well as the hormones that get rid of fat.

Just so you'll know, the micronutrients are vitamins, minerals, and trace elements. They provide no caloric energy, but they are necessary for life. Without the micronutrients we would suffer from deficiency diseases. Micronutrients are important too, but not as critical for reducing calories.

What is a calorie? It is a unit of energy. In the lab, a calorie is the amount of heat it takes to raise the temperature of one gram of water one degree Celsius. Most of us think of calories in terms of the number found on the back of a food label that can make us fat. While eating excessive calories can make you fat, understanding what calories do will make changing your body composition a lot easier.

Our bodies need energy to operate. From breathing to digesting food, to moving and exercising, the calories derived from food provide the fuel. Fat, carbohydrates, and protein all provide us with energy, but in different amounts. One gram of fat provides nine calories of energy; one gram of protein provides four calories of energy; and one gram of carbohydrate provides four calories of energy.

> **Dr. Z says . . .** *"You can do the math. Let's say a food contains 10 grams of carbs, 0 grams of protein, and 0 grams of fat per serving. That means it contains 40 calories (10 grams x 4 calories per gram = 40 calories). Now let's look at fat. If a food contains 0 grams of carbs, 0 grams of protein, and 10 grams of fat, that means it contains 90 calories (10 grams x 9 calories per gram = 90 calories)."*

Now that we know that, we should consider what each of these nutrients does. When you learn what you're putting into your body, you can make better decisions about what you want to buy at the store.

Carbohydrates (Carbs)

Carbohydrates are the macronutrient we need the most, because they are the cleanest burning in the body. They provide glucose, the main fuel for cells. Carbs also are needed for the brain and nervous system, the heart and muscular system, and for the kidneys. Carbs help to keep the intestines healthy, and they are stored in the liver and muscles for later use. The most common forms of carbs are starches, fibers, and sugars. These are grouped into two categories: simple and complex carbs. Examples of simple carbs are table sugar, fruit sugar, honey, and other sweets. Examples of complex carbs are brown rice, carrots, sweet potatoes, legumes, steel-cut oats, and brown-rice pasta.

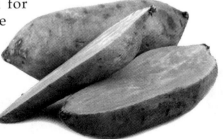

Drawing a distinction between simple and complex carbs is important. Too much misinformation has been passed around about carbs because many diet books treat the two as if they are the same. Carbohydrates are classified based on their chemical structure and how quickly they are digested and absorbed. Simple carbs like soda, cakes, cookies, pies, and candy are digested and absorbed quickly. That causes a fast rise in blood sugar. Simple carbs usually have no real nutrient value, as they lack vitamins and minerals. Complex carbs, also known as starches, are digested slowly and don't raise blood sugar quickly. As mentioned above, the best complex carbs are brown-rice pasta and steel-cut oats, as well as some vegetables like sweet potato, squash, and beets. They are packed with vitamins, minerals, and fiber. You can guess which type is best for your body composition.

Glucose, the body's key source of energy, comes from carbohydrates. Glucose is stored in the liver and turned into muscle energy called glycogen. Glucose is found in all the sugars we consume, including fructose (fruit sugar), sucrose (refined table sugar), and lactose (dairy sugar). However, the body uses these types of sugar in different ways.

Fructose is broken down in two ways. It either becomes glucose for energy, or it is converted to fatty acids, or fat. These fatty acids are turned into triglycerides and transported to the muscles and fat cells to make fat. The best type is natural fructose, which is found in plants—fruits, vegetables, and some legumes (beans). It is the best type because fructose naturally found in fruits and vegetables also contains fiber. According to the *Journal of Nutrition*, dietary fiber decreases the speed at which the body absorbs fructose. 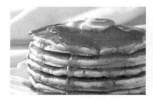 Decreasing the speed may help to prevent the highs and lows in blood sugar, reducing the risk for type 2 diabetes. It also will help to prevent you from getting fat.

Sucrose, or table sugar, is broken down by the body into glucose and fructose. The glucose is used for energy, and the fructose gets stored as fat. Diets high in refined sugars (table sugars and high-fructose corn syrup) will make you fat. High-fructose corn syrup is made from corn starch; the glucose part of the starch is chemically altered to produce refined fructose. Notice that I said "refined." That means it's not natural; it does not contain fiber. The processed-food industry uses it in breads, cereals, yogurts, soups, condiments, sodas, energy drinks, breakfast bars, lunchmeats, and just about any non-food "food" product.

Lactose, the sugar derived from milk products, is broken down into glucose and galactose. Galactose is then converted into glucose and stored in the liver. Lactose is familiar mainly because of "lactose intolerance," a common condition today. Lactose should not be consumed beyond infancy. If you are lactose intolerant, your body is telling you that you should not drink milk. Why is that? Milk is the food source for babies of a specific species. Human infants drink human breast milk; calves drink cow milk; and monkeys drink monkey milk. After weaning, when we no longer need to drink milk, the body stops producing the enzyme lactase, which is specifically created to break down milk sugar. We are genetically designed to stop producing lactase when we transition to solid food sources. So, if you have a reaction to dairy products, it's because your body can't break down the lactose. The milk sugar causes a reaction with the bacteria in your gut, causing bloating, pain, and diarrhea—creating the condition known as lactose intolerance. That "condition" is actually normal. Beyond infancy, we are not supposed to drink milk or eat foods containing milk. After all, do you know anyone who is water intolerant?

At our first discussion, Kirk C. handed me a huge folder loaded with test results. His complaint was abdominal bloating, pain, and diarrhea—which occurred eight times a day. He was afraid to leave the house, and his gut problem was affecting his job. He listed the tests done to identify his mysterious health problem. He'd had an endoscopy, colonoscopy, repeated blood work, barium studies of his stomach, stool (diarrhea) testing, and, last but not least, a biopsy of his intestine. He had agreed to all that testing out of a desperate hope of finding something to explain his misery. However, all the tests came back normal.

I then asked Kirk what he was eating. He stopped short, then said, "No doctor ever asked me that." My first thought was: Why the hell (I'm being nice here) was he not asked what he was eating? Diet and lifestyle are the most important factors in reversing and preventing disease. He told me his typical diet consisted of eggs and fruit in the morning, a sandwich and more fruit for lunch, and a variety of proteins with vegetables for dinner. He paused and added, "Oh, yeah, I eat a pint of Ben and Jerry's ice cream before bed."

Health problem solved. He had a simple case of lactose intolerance. Given the list of doctors he had seen, and the amount of testing they did, I was surprised that no one asked him the simple question of what he was eating. Kirk agreed to eliminate the dairy. I recommended he take digestive enzymes to help him with digestion, plus a multispectral probiotic to repopulate his gut with healthy bacteria. I changed his diet to include not just healthful proteins and carbs, but plenty of green vegetables and legumes (beans), which are all high in fiber. Eating this way helped to resolve the long-term inflammation he had in his gut due to the dairy products he was eating. In a few days, he had no more stomach troubles, and in less than three weeks, Kirk reported that he had more energy and felt the best he had in a long time.

I mentioned fiber before. Exactly what is that? Fiber is a type of carbohydrate that the body cannot digest. As fiber passes through the gut, it helps to remove waste from the body. You can think of it as a scrubber that works inside your tubes. A diet high in fiber helps to regulate blood fats, control blood sugars, and reduce inflammation. Foods high in fiber include fruits, vegetables, and whole-grain products.

Protein

Protein is the building block of life. When protein is digested, it breaks down into amino acids. These are classified as essential or nonessential, which is not as complicated as it sounds. The difference is that the body cannot make essential amino acids; they must be supplied by food. Protein is needed for all stages of life. It is needed for growth and development. It helps repair cells and tissues when they are damaged. It is also needed for muscles and bones, for creating hormones, and for the immune system to fight off infections. Examples of proteins include beef, bison, venison, chicken, turkey, fish, seafood, and eggs.

You may have heard of high-protein diets. What is the story with them? They are set up to promote high levels of protein. As a result, they cause a drastic reduction in carbohydrate consumption. When carbs are dramatically reduced from the diet, the body goes into a state called ketosis, where it burns fat for energy. Normally we get energy from carbs, but when there is no energy coming from carbs, fat is broken down into ketones, which then supply us with energy. As a result, you go from burning carbs for energy to burning fat for energy. According to the *American Journal of Clinical Nutrition*, high-protein, low-carb diets have been found to reduce hunger, decrease calorie consumption, and induce significant weight loss. Eating high amounts of protein causes a drop in the hormones that regulate appetite. So, when you eat more protein, you are less hungry. Therefore, you eat less. Yet there is a catch. Most diets that promote eating high protein and low carbs may cause potential health problems down the road.

Most high-protein diets don't permit a high intake of carbohydrates from fruits and starchy vegetables. By omitting those carbs from the diet, you risk not taking in enough B vitamins (including folate), vitamin C, and fiber. These nutrients are vital for your body. Those same high-protein diets also promote eating foods like dairy products, which may increase your risk for heart disease, autoimmune diseases, and certain cancers. Furthermore, individuals with kidney disease may have trouble eliminating the waste products of a protein-spurred metabolism. Yes, having more protein helps you lose fat. However, I don't agree with excluding carbs and other food sources, which provide vital nutrients. The trick here is to get rid of the fat with only short periods of ketosis. This is done by eating a variety of foods, including protein, fats, and carbs.

Finally, what about the folks promoting no-meat, no-fat diets? The theory that eating animal protein, and any kind of fat, will kill you does not line up with the facts or even common sense. Humans have been around for millions of years. According to the *Annual Review of Anthropology*, eating animal products and fat provided vital nutrients and polyunsaturated fats necessary for the development of a larger brain. Early humans ate fruits, vegetables, and tubers, but they were also scavengers, eating the leftover carcasses of animals killed by carnivores. Besides the leftover meat, they ate the brain and bone marrow of the animal, which provided them a source of fat for energy. In fact, eating the brains of animals provided early man with an omega-3 fatty acid called docosahexaenoic acid, or DHA, which is essential for the development of the brain and nervous system. Early humans got most of their energy from consuming super-lean meats, which also provided fat-soluble vitamins like A, D, E, and K. Animal meat, organs, and brains also provided early man with concentrated sources of iron, calcium, sodium, zinc, and B vitamins, including B1, niacin, B6, B12, and folate. Animal protein was, and is, needed for physical development and health. In *The Journal of Nutrition*, routine access to animal-source foods is the most likely reason behind our evolutionary development into large social beings.

Certain healthful, lean, free-range meats are loaded with omega-3 essential fatty acids and an abundance of nutrients that we need. These meats do not come, however, from abused livestock, injected with synthetic hormones to keep them lactating long after they give birth. Those animals are shot up with antibiotics and fed unnatural food sources such as grain—not grass, but cereal grains. Unfortunately, for most of us, our food supply is controlled by companies that put this crap into the meats. You need to buy free-range, grass-fed, organic meats that have no toxins, providing a healthful source of protein.

What about the fat-free part of the diet? As with many types of foods, you need to make distinctions between different types of fats. Olive oil is not the same as butter, or margarine, or partially hydrogenated vegetable oil, which is synthetically made in a processing plant. Unhealthful fake fats are hazardous to our health. In the next section I will

Z Note

Everyday toxins are a serious hazard. Many people unwittingly add a wide range of environmental toxins to their bodies, creating conditions that promote cancer, diabetes, obesity, and other chronic diseases. It's a well-known fact that pesticides and herbicides are sprayed on our produce; PCB's are found in the soil and water supply, along with dioxins, bisphenol A, and phthalates from plastic household products. These toxins have been shown to damage cellular DNA, destroy the immune system, promote tumor growth, and make cancers more aggressive. These chemicals are also commonly referred to as endocrine disruptors; they interfere with the hormonal system and thus produce adverse reproductive, developmental, and neurological effects.

The *American Journal of Epidemiology* and *Advances in Breast Cancer Research* found the common organochlorine pesticide DDT (dichlorodiphenyltrichloroethane) and the environmental toxin PCB (polychlorinated biphenyl) to be carcinogenic. The researchers found these chemicals acted as weak estrogen, which made cancers of the breast and prostate more aggressive.

Obesity is now a global problem, not only for individuals, but also for the healthcare system and the economy. High-calorie, low nutrient-dense foods, combined with a lack of physical activity, represent the major cause of this pandemic. However, recent findings published in the journals *Endocrinology* and *Environmental Health Perspectives* have found a third culprit behind the obesity issue. They report that endocrine disruptors like DDT, bisphenol A (BPA), PCB, organotins, etc., can increase the number and size of fat cells, and alter the hormones involved in appetite, satiety, and food preferences. In combination with processed foods and physical inactivity, these obesogens (chemicals that make more fat) are becoming a major factor in the development of obesity.

Endocrine disruptors and obesogens may be found in everyday products, including plastic bottles, metal food cans, detergents, flame-retardants, food, toys, cosmetics, and pesticides. To help reduce the burden of toxins that you ingest, as well as their potential health risks, consider buying organic produce from your local farmers and farm stands. Second, clean your produce with a vegetable-and-fruit wash. You may also want to look for household products that are free of BPA, phthalate, and dioxins. Not only are these chemicals hazardous to bugs, they pose a real threat to us.

show you what the difference is between healthful fats and hazardous fats.

Fats

Fats come in solid form, such as avocado, or liquid form, such as olive oil. Fats provide us with essential fatty acids—the type that must come from food. Fats are needed for growth and development, as well as maintenance of healthy cell membranes. Fats provide cushioning for the organs and are needed for the body to absorb the fat-soluble vitamins A, D, E, and K. Some examples of liquid fats include fish oils, olive oil, grapeseed oil, avocado oil, coconut oil, and ghee (from butter). Solid forms include animal fats, avocado, nuts, nut butters, and seeds.

Understanding why some fats are good or bad for you will help you lose weight. The first way to break them down is to categorize fats as saturated or unsaturated. Saturated fats are "saturated" with hydrogen atoms, while unsaturated fats have few hydrogen atoms. Most saturated fats are solid at room temperature, and unsaturated fats are liquid at room temperature. Animal fats are saturated; they include cream, butter, cheese, ghee, lard, eggs, and meats. A few vegetable products, such as coconut oil, palm kernel oil, and chocolate, also contain saturated fats.

Unsaturated fats are broken down further into two categories: monounsaturated or polyunsaturated. Monounsaturated fats are found in nuts and nut oils, olives and olive oil, grapeseed oil, oatmeal, and avocados. Polyunsaturated fats contain omega-3, omega-6, and omega-9 fatty acids. Polyunsaturated fats are found in nuts, seeds, fish (sardines, tuna, wild salmon), olive oil, seaweed, green leafy vegetables, and algae.

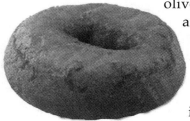

While both saturated and unsaturated fats have health benefits, the fats to avoid absolutely are trans fats. Those are fats used in food processing. The chemical processing of a trans fat is known as hydrogenation, or partial hydrogenation. Partially hydrogenated fats are toxic and dangerous. They are found in snack foods, baked goods, deep-fried foods, and fast foods, specifically junk vegetable oils, shortening, margarine, French fries, fried chicken, chicken nuggets, chips, taco shells, doughnuts, pizza dough, hot chocolate mixes, croutons, salad dressings, crackers, cookies, pastries, and breadcrumbs . . . to name a few. Junk-food companies use partially hydrogenated fats because they are less prone to going bad or rancid, which allows for a longer shelf life. Eating foods with a long shelf life may shorten your shelf life.

Let's say you took a bottle of corn oil, which is unsaturated, and you wanted to turn it into margarine, which is a solid. Through this chemical process called hydrogenation, you would add hydrogen atoms to the oil, which would make it partially hydrogenated. Partially hydrogenated vegetable oil is the main ingredient in margarine and vegetable shortening. Why is this bad?

Partially hydrogenated fats, or trans fats, have been shown to lower HDL, the protein that carts fat out of the heart, and increase LDL, the protein that delivers fat to the heart. A high LDL has been associated with an increased risk for cardiovascular disease. Hydrogenated fats increase Lipoprotein (a), which is a heart disease marker that can increase inflammation and blood clotting, which are both associated with heart attacks and strokes. Trans fats also increase the risk for cancer, Alzheimer's disease, obesity, and diabetes. Now you can see why I include health along with losing weight. When you are eating healthfully, you will naturally keep off the weight.

Karen M. originally came to see me for treatment for dizziness, high cholesterol, and a high LDL level. After putting her on a lifestyle-change program, Karen's blood fats returned to normal levels, and she was very pleased. After several months, though, she returned in a panic. "Dr. Z, my cholesterol and LDL levels are high again. Now what?" After questioning her about changes in her lifestyle, she said, "I fell off the wagon and am eating sugar again—cookies, cakes, pies, and ice cream." I questioned her about why she went to the dark side, and her response was, "I was getting away with it. I know it's unhealthy, but I continued to binge anyway. I wasn't feeling bad, so I continued to eat junk, even though I know it's bad for me." She makes an interesting point. This sums up the mind-set many people have when they are eating just for taste. Maybe we feel immortal; we push our health limits until we're sick and dying. Is this not like a child pushing his/her boundaries until they are set, until there is some consequence?

Knowing that high-sugar, refined junk caused her blood fats to elevate, Karen eagerly got back to healthful eating. Her foods consisted of protein and healthful fats, as well as green and rainbow-colored vegetables. While she craved the processed simple sugars, we substituted healthful low-sugar fruits and starchy vegetables. Over the next couple of months, Karen's sugar cravings disappeared, and her cholesterol and LDL levels went back to normal.

Then and Now: How Our Diet Has Changed

Ample research shows that a poor diet—one consisting of processed, nutrient-deprived foods—is a major contributor, if not the leading contributor, to the rise in chronic disease and death in the United States. Heart disease, cancer, and type 2 diabetes, as well as conditions like high blood pressure, arthritis, and autoimmune disorders, are the end result of eating the Standard American Diet (SAD). This typically is made up of processed "meats," white sugar, dairy, and refined grains.

Let's go back in time for a moment and discuss how this contemporary diet is vastly different from the diet of our prehistoric ancestors. The foods consumed in the past were unprocessed and, until fire was discovered, were eaten raw. The *European Journal of Clinical Nutrition* describes our ancestral menu as consisting of vegetables, fruits, roots, herbs, insects, different meat sources, and fish. In addition to organs and muscle tissue, the bone marrow was eaten and bones were gnawed. This so-called "primitive" diet was nutrient dense and unprocessed.

Fast-forwarding to the present, food processing was developed. That involved the milling of grains, refinement of sugar, and canning of foods. These methods caused a significant loss of nutrients in those foods. Knowing this, companies decided to "enrich" and "fortify" foods, which added back certain nutrients. Recently, processed food companies decided to introduce synthetic chemicals in order to make foods glow, prevent spoilage, and make them addictive. The consequence of these artificial food chemicals is ill health. Why would you eat anything that says "artificial" on the label?

How does all of this relate to disease? Simply put, the consumption of processed foods works contrary to your genes—your DNA. The nutrients that come from unprocessed, whole foods—our prehistoric diet—act as information that talks to the genes, which regulate cell, tissue, and organ function. Without this information (consisting of vitamins, minerals, and phytochemicals) our cells, tissues, and organs begin to malfunction. This is called subclinical nutrient deficiency, which happens before symptoms occur. The longer you are nutrient starved, the worse the tissue dysfunction becomes; eventually the cells, tissues, and organs become diseased and fail. The end result is heart disease, cancer, type 2 diabetes, high blood pressure, autoimmune disease, arthritis, and/or obesity.

By contrast, in recent years extensive research has focused on disease control and prevention through the use of whole foods and the phytochemicals that are naturally found in them.

Eating whole foods, found in nature, provides us with all the nutrients that allow us to run disease free, and to age without crippling conditions and premature death. This brings up the food source that should never be referred to as a side dish at dinner.

I Lost 30 Pounds and Reduced My Cardiovascular Risk

John C. is a 47-year-old man with a busy life, juggling four children and a demanding career. While becoming successful in business and helping to raise a family, he neglected to focus on his health. When John was a child, his father suddenly died from a heart attack in front of him on the beach. For years the passing of his father haunted him, and he feared a sudden heart attack would happen to him at an early age. A couple of years ago, John began pursuing tests to rule in or rule out coronary-artery disease. He had the standard blood tests, stress tests, and calcium-score testing. His calcium score, cholesterol level, and blood sugar were all high. He realized he was developing coronary-artery disease, and the race was on to stop the disease. John did his research and became educated on the causes of heart disease, along with the lifestyle and diet changes that were needed to stop its progression. His fear motivated John to change his diet the best he knew. He began searching for someone who could offer the right solution, but also work with him long term to see him through it all. John was referred to me for nutritional advice and counseling. After reviewing his previous lab work, we decided to get more in-depth testing done. The results indicated insulin resistance and continued high blood sugar. In addition, his cholesterol, LDL, Apolipoprotein B, oxidized LDL, and C-reactive protein (CRP, an inflammatory marker) were also high.

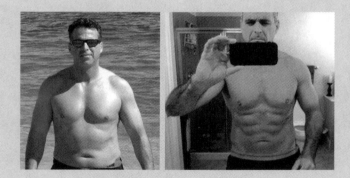

Before / After

John also complained of feeling soft, and hated the excess body fat he was carrying. When discussing his diet, I realized that he was eating processed, nutrient-void foods that consisted of white pastas, dairy, and too many sugary high-calorie foods. Also, he was not eating nearly enough plant-based foods to sustain normal function and reduce inflammation—the culprit behind coronary-artery disease. John became a soldier committed to seeing his condition improve. In the weeks following the elimination of refined grains, dairy, and white sugar, John never felt better. His body-fat percentage dropped dramatically, and he soon was staring at a six-pack he had once admired in college. Follow-up blood work confirmed that John's diet and lifestyle changes were paying off. His CRP is now normal, having dropped from 5.4 to .6, and the oxidized LDL is back to normal. Shortly, you will discover the role of oxidized LDL in coronary-artery disease.

The Power of Fruits and Vegetables

No other food source is more important for your health than plant-based foods. For years you have heard how important it is to eat plenty of fruits and vegetables, but with few reasons why. To start, fruits and vegetables are very low in calories and fat. They are loaded with antioxidants, enzymes, and phytochemicals, and also provide important vitamins. These include vitamins A, C, K, and E, as well as vitamins B1 (thiamine), B2 (riboflavin), B6, folate, pantothenic acid, and niacin. The minerals contained in fruits and vegetables include potassium, phosphorous, magnesium, sodium, calcium, iodine, iron, zinc, copper, manganese, and selenium. These vitamins and minerals help to run intricate cellular machinery responsible for producing energy, burning fat, detoxifying, and healing, as well as maintaining pH, electrolyte balance, nerve and muscle function, cellular repair, and proper immune function—to name a few.

I think it's important to mention some of the vitamins, minerals, and phytochemicals found in plant-based foods, as well as why eating them will not only help to get rid of your body fat. They can help you to rebuild your health, and prevent and reverse disease. Before I discuss the different vitamins, minerals, and phytonutrients found in plant-based foods, allow me to provide a definition for each. Vitamins are organic compounds required in limited amounts, which can't be made in the body; therefore, we need to get them through diet. Vitamins can act as coenzymes in metabolic reactions, and are effective antioxidants to combat free radicals. Minerals are inorganic compounds that serve as cofactors in enzymatic reactions, and they are constituents of hormones, proteins, and vitamins. Last, phytochemicals are plant compounds other than vitamins and minerals; they give fruits and vegetables their color and smell. Examples include the deep purple of blueberries, the brilliant orange of carrots or sweet potatoes, and the smell of garlic.

Vitamins are classified as either water-soluble or fat-soluble. Water-soluble vitamins dissolve in water and are not stored in the body; therefore, they must be taken in daily. The water-soluble vitamins include the family of B vitamins and vitamin C. In contrast, fat-soluble vitamins dissolve in fat before they are absorbed into the bloodstream. The fat-soluble vitamins are A, D, E, and K; they are stored in the liver.

Vitamin A

There are three forms of vitamin A—retinol, retinal, and retinoic acid—primarily found in animal-based foods, including liver and fish. Plant-based foods contain beta-carotene, an antioxidant that is converted into vitamin A. Vitamin A is important for immune function and good vision. It is also important for red-blood-cell production, gene expression, bone health, suppression of cancer, and normal iron metabolism. A deficiency in vitamin A can cause night blindness, a condition where your eyes cannot adjust to dim light. Vitamin-A deficiency can also cause thick and scaly skin, as well as sterility.

Foods abundant in beta-carotene include butternut squash, carrots, collards, kale, pumpkin, red pepper, spinach, and sweet potato.

B Vitamins

The family of B vitamins assists the body in making energy from the foods you eat. B vitamins are also needed for maintaining a normal appetite, good vision, healthy skin, smoothly running neurological function, and red-blood-cell formation. There are eight B vitamins in the B-complex group: B1 (thiamin), B2 (riboflavin), B3 (niacin), B5 (pantothenic acid), B6 (pyridoxine), folate, biotin, and B12 (cobalamin).

All B vitamins are involved in producing energy; however, each one has unique properties that are important to mention. In addition to energy production, thiamin supports the activity of nerves and muscles, including the heart. Inadequate thiamin levels can cause muscle weakness, pins-and-needles sensations, and numbness in the legs.

Riboflavin helps to protect from oxygen damage and is needed for detoxification. A deficiency can cause itching and burning around the mouth, sensitivity to light, peripheral neuropathy, soreness of the tongue, migraine headaches, and seborrheic dermatitis.

Niacin can help to lower blood fats and stabilize your blood sugar. Pellagra is the name of a collective group of symptoms that are a classic sign of a significant niacin deficiency: dermatitis, dementia, and dysentery (severe diarrhea).

Pantothenic acid (B5) helps your ability to respond to stress. If you are fatigued, weak, and depressed, or suffer from insomnia, you may have a vitamin B5 deficiency.

Pyridoxine (B6) is important for the breakdown of starches and prevents the buildup of homocysteine in the blood. Homocysteine is a compound linked to atherosclerosis and coronary-artery disease. B6 is also important in the prevention of anemia.

Folate—not folic acid, which is synthetic and not found in nature—supports healthy red blood cells, allows for proper nerve function, and prevents the birth defect spina bifida. Low folate levels can also cause elevated homocysteine and significant anemia.

Biotin is needed for healthy hair and skin. Alopecia is hair loss caused by multiple metabolic issues. One type is male-pattern baldness due to an excess of testosterone and dihydrotestosterone (DHT). A hypothyroid condition can also cause hair loss. If those aren't the reasons for the thinning hair, think biotin deficiency.

Last, there is vitamin B12. Cobalamin allows nerves to develop properly and helps you metabolize protein, carbs, and fats. It is needed for red blood cell formation, and it reduces the buildup of homocysteine.

Vitamin B12 is different from the other B vitamins; for proper absorption, it needs a ride into the small intestine from a protein called the intrinsic factor. While the other B vitamins are found in plant-based foods, B12 is found only in foods of animal origin, such as liver, meat, kidney, fish, shellfish, and eggs. B12 deficiency is often seen in strict vegetarians, the elderly, infants of vegan mothers, and autoimmune disorders where the immune system targets the intrinsic factor. A B12 deficiency causes fatigue, anemia, nerve damage, numbness and tingling in the limbs, dementia, and a loss of memory. This collective list of symptoms is called pernicious anemia.

Now that you know more about the B vitamins, their functions, benefits, and signs of deficiencies, you need to know where to find them. Asparagus, avocado, beans, bell peppers, broccoli, brown rice, dark-green leafy vegetables, eggplant, green peas, lentils, mushrooms, squash, Swiss chard, tomatoes, wheat germ, and whole grains are all good sources of B vitamins, with the exception of B12, which, again, is found only in animal-based foods.

Risky Procedures

An important fact for those who have gone through gastric-bypass surgery, or are considering having it done, is that gastric bypass causes significant malabsorption of vitamin B12. If you are not familiar with the surgery, here is a quick overview. During normal digestion the food passes from the stomach into the small intestine, where nutrients are absorbed. As digestion continues, the broken-down food passes into the large intestine (colon), and waste is eventually eliminated. Gastric-bypass surgery radically changes the way you digest your food and absorb nutrients.

The most common gastric-bypass procedure is called the Roux-en-Y gastric bypass, whereby the lower part of the stomach is "rearranged" surgically into a Y configuration: the stomach is divided into a large portion and a much smaller portion (the size of an egg). This smaller part is "stapled" into a little pouch and connected directly to the middle of the small intestine, bypassing the upper portion. The larger, leftover part of the stomach is then disconnected from the small intestine. The end result is a much smaller stomach, which forces you to eat less and feel less hungry.

According to the *Annals of Surgery*, following the Roux-en-Y gastric bypass, stomach-acid secretion is virtually absent, and food-bound vitamin B12 is maldigested and malabsorbed. The fact that stomach-acid secretion is virtually absent following the bypass is a very serious issue. For one, protein digestion happens in the stomach; without acid there is improper protein breakdown and absorption. Without protein, the body and all of its intricate systems begin to fail. Stomach acid is also a disinfectant. By shutting off its production, there is a risk of developing gut infections, such as Helicobacter (H. Pylori) and Vibrio. An undetected and untreated H. Pylori infection is associated with a high risk of lymphoma, a type of cancer, in the gut.

Moreover, if you don't stop eating processed foods, making your stomach smaller is a temporary Band-Aid. High-calorie foods will continue to flip the fat-storing switches regardless of how small the stomach becomes. Therefore, if you deprive yourself of nutrients by choice—a poor diet—or it is forced through invasive procedures, you increase your risk for chronic disease.

Jamie B. is a 21-year-old cancer victor who struggled with her body composition for years. Following surgery to remove a tumor within her brain, radiation was used to ensure the cancer was destroyed. Unfortunately, the damage it caused created abnormal hormone levels, altered metabolism, and created extreme weight gain. For years she tried to control her weight through proper food choices and exercise, but the fight got to be too much. Jamie finally opted for gastric-bypass surgery. Two years following the surgery, she, accompanied by her mom, scheduled a visit with me to discuss possible treatment options for current problems. Not long after the surgery, she had begun suffering from chronic headaches and fatigue, which became progressively worse with time. In tears, Jamie said she was unable to have a social life, or go out and enjoy herself, because she had developed chronic diarrhea that occurred every time she took a bite of food. To add to her misery, she was also dealing with a viral infection, which was probably adding to her fatigue.

Upon reviewing her blood work, I saw clearly the long-term effects of the surgery. Vitamin B12 and iron were not being absorbed, which created a severe anemia. Her blood work revealed a low red blood cell count, low hemoglobin and hematocrit, and extremely low iron levels. The unrelenting diarrhea was caused by abnormal stomach-acid production and improper breakdown of her food. The immediate plan was to stop the diarrhea. I gave her digestive enzymes to be taken every time she had a bite of food. After the first time she used the enzymes, her diarrhea stopped. The next obstacle was to help her to digest and absorb vitamin B12 and iron. She started a scientifically formulated multivitamin with iron and a special B-vitamin complex. I encouraged her to take the enzymes when she ate any meat in order to break down the protein and facilitate B12 absorption. At her next visit, new blood work revealed improvements in her anemia, including higher red-blood-cell count, hemoglobin, hematocrit, iron, and ferritin (iron storage).

Having your stomach cut open and rearranged doesn't sound like a safe diet choice. Gastric-bypass surgery is a major surgery with long-term health consequences. If you know someone considering this procedure, please show them this book and encourage them to read and apply the tools within. The only side effect of the Body Composition Diet is a low-fat and healthy body.

Vitamin C

Of all the vitamins essential to our health, vitamin C (ascorbic acid) is at the top of the list. Why? Because it is not made in the body, it has to be taken in through the diet, thus making it essential. It is also a powerful antioxidant, important for building and maintaining healthy tissue through collagen synthesis. Vitamin C helps to maintain healthy teeth and gums, promotes antibody production, and is needed for iron absorption. Last, vitamin C supports detoxification, increases HDL production, and is needed for the excretion or elimination of heavy metals.

Coronary-artery disease is still the number-one killer on the planet, despite cholesterol-lowering drugs, stents, and bypass surgery. Current research states that coronary-artery disease (CAD) is not a consequence of cholesterol sticking to and clogging the arteries. Research clearly states that CAD is an inflammatory condition within the wall of the artery. Simply put, coronary-artery disease develops in stages:

1. Due to a number of reasons—smoking, junk food, consuming partially hydrogenated vegetable oil, or having high blood pressure—the endothelium (a single-celled layer lining the inside of the artery) becomes damaged. This allows the passage of low-density lipoprotein (LDL) and white blood cells into the wall of the artery.

2. LDL brings cholesterol into the arterial wall, where it is oxidized or damaged by free radicals. White blood cells, called macrophages, recognize the oxidized LDL and proceed to gobble up the LDL along with its cholesterol.

3. After consuming the damaged LDL, the macrophages turn into foam cells, which spit out inflammatory chemicals and enzymes, causing swelling and damage to the protective layers of cells in the wall. This swelling and damage is called a vulnerable plaque.

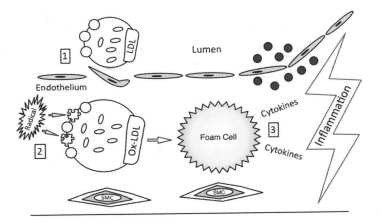

Eventually the damage within the arterial wall causes an eruption of material and debris within the lumen (opening of the artery), quickly shutting off the blood supply to the heart muscle, leading to a sudden heart attack (myocardial infarct).

According to the *Bratislava Medical Journal,* vitamin C (ascorbic acid) protects LDL from oxidation. The researchers found that carotid-artery disease is less pronounced in men with high blood levels of vitamin C. They also found that in parts of Western Europe, deaths from cardiovascular causes fell rapidly following a movement to increase intake of vitamin C. Conversely, cardiovascular deaths are still growing in those areas with known vitamin-C deficiency.

In reading through hundreds of research articles involving the mechanism of coronary-artery disease, I saw that a major step in the process is the oxidation of LDL. Vitamin C protects LDL from oxidation. In a research article published in the *New England Journal of Medicine,* subjects whose vitamin-C intake exceeded 50 mg per day had a lower rate of death from all cardiovascular disease. Getting more than 50 mg per day is pretty easy; for instance, one kiwi provides 84 mg of vitamin C, while broccoli provides 81 mg of vitamin C per cup, chopped. If you have four to five servings of fruits and vegetables a day, that will provide enough vitamin C to prevent heart disease.

What about cancer? Since cancer was close to my heart, literally, I will point out the benefits of vitamin C in staving off cancer. It is a well-known fact that, under sustained environmental stress, free radicals are produced in the body over a long time. These free radicals can damage the DNA of the cells, which may cause the initial mutations within the cell. The DNA and genetic code within those cells multiply and divide out of control until they become a detectable cancerous tumor. The National Cancer Institute recommends five servings a day of plant-based foods—vegetables and fruits—that lower your risk for cancers of the mouth, throat, stomach, lung, colon, pancreas, and prostate.

Vitamin C is readily available in citrus fruits (lemon, lime, grapefruit, orange, and tangerine), as well as broccoli, Brussels sprouts, cauliflower, kale, kiwi, red and green peppers, strawberries, and sweet potato. Other food sources with vitamin C include apple, black currants, cabbage, cantaloupe, guava, honeydew melon, mango, mustard greens, papaya, raspberries, red and green hot chili peppers, and spinach.

> ## Z Note
>
> Oxidation takes place when free radicals attack and damage the LDL particle; think of hail from a storm denting the hood of a car. A common theme, threaded throughout the research, states that free radicals from a processed and nutrient-deprived diet, high blood sugar, and smoking are the initiators and main drivers for this preventable, lifestyle-based, and often fatal disease.

Vitamin D: A Powerful Hormone

You may be wondering why I didn't include vitamin D in the original list of nutrients found in plant-based foods. First, although it is called a vitamin, vitamin D is actually a hormone. Vitamins are obtained through diet, not made in the body, unlike hormones, which are made in the body. There are two forms of vitamin D: D2 is found in fungi, like mushrooms, but not found in green leafy plants. D3 is generated when your skin is exposed to UV radiation from sunlight. D3 is also found in oily fish, cod-liver oil, herring, mackerel, salmon, sardines, tuna, and, to a lesser extent, egg yolks.

The classic manifestation of vitamin-D deficiency in children is rickets, while in adults it causes osteomalacia (softening of the bones). However, low levels of vitamin D have been implicated in almost every major disease, including:

+ Osteoporosis
+ Cancer
+ Heart disease
+ Autoimmune disease
+ High blood pressure
+ Infertility
+ Depression
+ Chronic pain
+ Psoriasis

How is vitamin D made? After sunlight comes in contact with the skin, the body produces a chemical that travels to the liver then to the kidneys to become the active form of vitamin D called calcitriol. This helps the intestine absorb calcium, and maintains normal calcium and phosphate levels for bone formation. It enhances muscle strength, has anti-inflammatory effects, and regulates the immune system. Calcitriol also helps to control cell growth, which researchers have found can prevent cancer.

With the patients who come to see me about unresolved health issues, I often see common threads. One is a nutrient-deprived diet, and the other is a low level of vitamin D. One major cause of that is the fear of skin cancer, which has driven people to avoid the sun. Yet melanoma (a deadly form of skin cancer) is usually not located on parts of the body that get sun exposure. *The Journal of Skin Cancer* found that, although outdoor workers get three to ten times the annual dose of UV radiation that indoor workers get, they—outdoor workers—have similar or lower incidents of malignant melanoma. The human race has been out in the sun for millions of years, yet we are still around.

Z Note

Stephen R. is a fair-skinned man who is speckled with birthmarks. His job keeps him indoors, and he doesn't find much time for the sun. Doing the responsible thing, Steve was getting his birthmarks checked by a dermatologist for 15 years. He was aware of a strange mark on his inner thigh, but his dermatologist told him the mark/ mole was not skin cancer. However, it was eventually revealed to be melanoma. The skin cancer had progressed long enough to metastasize into the lymph nodes of his leg. He and the oncologist acted right away by removing all the diseased lymph nodes in the leg, along with the removal of the original cancer site. The oncologist had no other recommendation for him except to start chemotherapy, which is known to be ineffective against metastatic melanoma. At Steve's first visit with me, the swelling in his leg was significant. He came to me looking for nutritional information to help him heal and to find out if there was some unknown reason for his condition. His history revealed little time outside due to his job, a processed diet, and, as expected, low vitamin-D levels.

You may have thought that vitamin D is also important for the health of bones, and you're right. Vitamin D is needed to absorb calcium from foods, which is used to build healthy bones and teeth. Not only is it responsible for the absorption of calcium, vitamin D is also important for bone mineralization, a process of adding calcium to the matrix of bones in order to make them hard and durable. Recalling rickets and osteomalacia, it is evident that demineralized and deformed bones are due to severe vitamin-D deficiency.

A common and often disabling condition of the bones usually seen in the elderly is osteoporosis. In that condition, bone-mineral density is reduced and the bone architecture breaks down, creating empty and weak bones. Usually happening in women after menopause, osteoporosis increases risk of fractures of the spinal bones and of the long bones and hips. Fractures of the spine lead to the stooped posture that appears as a flexed hunchback. These spinal-compression fractures are often very painful. Fractures of the hip are not only immobilizing, they can be life threatening. The risk associated with hip fractures is deep-vein thrombosis (a blood clot from the veins of the leg), which can cause a pulmonary embolus (blockage of a main artery in the lung), which, in turn, can cause sudden death. Need I say more? Vitamin D is essential for bone health, and a deficiency of vitamin D can contribute to osteoporosis.

What about the relationship between vitamin D and body composition? An article published in the *Nutrition Journal* showed evidence that taking a supplement with vitamin D and calcium helped to get rid of body fat. The study was conducted with two groups. One group went on a calorie-restrictive diet of only 500 calories per day. The second group also reduced their calorie intake to 500 calories a day, but also supplemented daily with vitamin D and calcium. Both groups followed the diet through the study for 12 weeks. At the end of the study, the group taking the supplement of vitamin D and calcium showed a significant decrease in fat mass over the group who followed the calorie-restrictive diet alone.

In addition, population studies are revealing the relationship between grain/bread consumption and low levels of vitamin D. In "Cereal Grains: Humanity's Double-Edged Sword," an article in *The World Review of Nutrition and Dietetics*, it was found that whole-grain cereal products impair bone metabolism by limiting calcium intake and altering vitamin-D metabolism. Population studies are also showing a widespread vitamin-D deficiency in people who consume whole-grain breads. That's not counting the fact that the majority of grains eaten are refined—white and even most "whole wheat" flour. If whole grains are depleting our vitamin-D levels, what's the processed stuff doing to us?

Z Note

The research on vitamin D is extraordinary. Facts found in the journal *Nature Reviews* found that calcitriol—the active form of vitamin D—had multiple effects on cancer. Calcitriol was shown to inhibit abnormal cellular growth and decrease the spread of cancer. It also turned on a program in the cancer cells that causes them to commit suicide. Last, in order for cancer cells and tumors to survive, they must create their own blood supply to provide nutrients and sugar. This process is known as angiogenesis. Calcitriol was shown to inhibit angiogenesis, thus starving cancer of its lifeline of nutrients.

Most of these studies have reported that higher blood levels of vitamin D are associated with lower rates of breast, colon, ovarian, kidney, pancreatic, prostate, and other cancers. Evidence found in the journal *Annals of Epidemiology* was alarming. It was projected that raising the year-round levels of vitamin D from 30 ng/ml to 40 to 60 ng/ml in the blood would prevent approximately 58,000 new cases of breast cancer and 49,000 new cases of colorectal cancer each year, in addition to preventing three-fourths of the deaths from those cancers. This is unheard of. By raising the levels of vitamin D beyond the "standards of care," thousands of people would be spared the emotional and physical devastation of cancer diagnosis and treatment, and their lives could be saved.

Finally, research is also discovering the relationship between cardiovascular disease and low vitamin-D levels. The *Journal of Invasive Cardiology* reported that patients with lower vitamin-D levels had a higher number of double- or triple-vessel coronary-artery disease and diffuse coronary-artery disease. Those with low vitamin-D levels also exhibited dysfunction of the endothelium—the cells that line and protect the arteries, help to regulate blood pressure, and protect against atherosclerosis and coronary-artery disease.

Clinical Note

A test to measure the amount of vitamin D in your blood is the only way to know if you are getting enough vitamin D from the sun and/or supplements you may be taking. The blood test you need is the 25(OH)D. The optimal range for vitamin D levels is 50 to 80 ng/ml, not 30 ng/ml—the standard.

Vitamin E

The next fat-soluble vitamin abundant in vegetables is vitamin E, another antioxidant that helps to prevent cell damage and plays a major role in protecting LDL from being damaged by free radicals. Vitamin E keeps the immune system in proper working order and helps to reduce the proliferation of cells. It is considered the fertility-E vitamin, since studies have revealed its importance to reproductive health. A deficiency of vitamin E is characterized by muscle and nervous-system disorders, cataracts, hemolytic anemia (red-blood-cell destruction), reproductive disorders (including a thin uterine lining), decreased sperm motility, and miscarriages.

Vitamin E is found in almonds, asparagus, avocado, beet greens, broccoli, collard greens, dandelion greens, dark-green leafy vegetables, hazelnuts, pumpkin, sunflower seeds, sweet potato, turnips, and healthful vegetable oils, including olive and wheat-germ oil.

Vitamin K for K-oagulation

Vitamin K is the last of the fat-soluble vitamins. There are two forms of vitamin K: K1 from green plants and K2 from bacteria in the intestines. It is needed for healthy bones; however, the biggest role of vitamin K is in blood clotting. The best food sources of vitamin K1 are dark-green leafy vegetables such as cabbage, lettuce, spinach, and turnip greens.

Z Note

Vitamin K deficiency is caused by a poor diet, and some pharmaceuticals, such as anti-clotting medications (Coumadin, warfarin), as well as broad-spectrum antibiotics (amoxicillin, streptomycin, tetracycline).

Minerals for Optimal Health

Along with vitamins, the minerals found in foods control and regulate reactions in the body. We cannot create minerals; therefore, we must get them from the foods we eat—both plant- and animal-based. Plants absorb minerals from the soil, and we get most of our minerals from the plants we eat. We also get minerals from animal foods, as they also get minerals from the plants they eat.

Calcium

Calcium is important for blood clotting and the passage of nutrients through cell walls, and it is essential for strong bones and teeth. As a dynamic "live" tissue, bone is constantly undergoing remodeling and turnover. Bone cells are constantly building and breaking down. This remodeling is essential to bone health and depends on calcium intake. It is needed also for muscle contraction and to help nerves carry messages.

A deficiency of calcium may result in muscle cramps, poor nerve firing, and bone demineralization or osteoporosis. Calcium-rich foods include: beans, broccoli, Brussels sprouts, butternut squash, dark leafy greens, kale, spinach, Swiss chard, and turnips. For the most part, any vegetable matter that can be eaten provides calcium. Fruits with calcium are blackberries, black currents, dates, grapefruit, orange, and pomegranate. Calcium is also found in eggs, perch, pollack, and sardines.

Not seeing milk here? Read why on page 87 of the section called "Our Worst Friends" later in this chapter for more information on calcium and milk.

Copper

Copper in small amounts is essential for the absorption and storage of iron and the formation of red blood cells, among other functions. It also helps to regulate blood sugar and immune function. Copper deficiency shows up in anemia, low white-blood-cell count, skeletal demineralization, poor wound healing, and weak muscles.

Copper-abundant foods include: artichoke, avocado, beans, beef, blackberries, dates, kiwi, mango, nuts, parsnip, peas, potatoes, pumpkin, salmon, sardines, squash, sunflower seeds, sweet potato, Swiss chard, and turkey.

Z Note

A deficiency of copper may be a causative factor in congestive heart failure and an enlarged heart. A study published in the *European Heart Journal* found that those with chronic heart failure and ischemic heart disease had an improvement in heart function while taking a copper supplement. In addition to this study, there are multiple animal studies that show that a copper deficiency in animals can induce cardiac enlargement and heart failure that are reversible with copper supplementation.

Iodine: The Th-i-roid Nutrient

Iodine is a mineral that is abundant in seaweed and other edible plants from the sea. Iodine helps to regulate energy production, and it promotes healthy skin, nails, and teeth. Its biggest role is to provide normal function to the thyroid. The thyroid gland, seated in your upper throat, uses iodine to produce the hormones T3 and T4 that regulate the way we metabolize carbohydrates, protein, and fats, thus making them very important to a healthy body composition.

When iodine is deficient in the diet, we develop hypothyroidism, a condition where the thyroid produces too little of the thyroid hormones T3 and T4. Lack of iodine also increases the risk of certain cancers, including cancer of the thyroid, breast, and prostate. Ironically, food companies know that processed foods have no nutritional value, so they add iodine to salt. The problem is that most iodized table salt is processed and is missing over 80 minerals found in natural salt.

You should avoid all processed flours found in baked goods (bread, cakes, muffins, bagels, etc.), because the bromide found in refined flour displaces iodine.

Iron

Iron is an essential mineral needed for the formation of hemoglobin, a protein that carries oxygen in the blood to tissues and organs of the body. It also brings carbon dioxide back to the lungs for elimination. Iron is also needed for the formation of myoglobin, which carries oxygen to the muscles. It is also needed for energy production, neurotransmitter production, and the immune system.

There are two forms of iron: heme iron and non-heme iron. Heme iron is found in clams, fish, meats, oysters, and poultry and is well absorbed. Non-heme iron is poorly absorbed and found in dried apricots, bok choy, broccoli, Brussels sprouts, dark-green vegetables, grains, kale, legumes (beans), millet, nuts, quinoa, sesame seeds, Swiss chard, and turnip greens. Fortunately, plant-based foods also provide vitamin C, which promotes iron absorption.

Iron is the most common mineral deficiency, which, according to the Centers for Disease Control and Prevention, is the leading cause of anemia in the United States. Iron deficiency is caused by either an increased need for iron, poor absorption, or a diet lacking in iron. Those at greatest risk for iron deficiency are infants, pregnant women, and adolescent girls. Infants and the young need more iron because they are rapidly growing. Menstruation increases the demand for iron due to blood loss. Iron needs increase during pregnancy due to the fetal requirements. Vegans are at risk for iron deficiency because their diets do not include heme iron. Those with internal bleeding disorders, including ulcers, colon cancer, and ulcerative colitis, are also at risk.

The effects of iron deficiency can include abnormal behavior, impaired mental cognition, impaired immune function, fatigue, weakness, problems regulating body temperature, and angular stomatitis—fissures or cracking of the skin at the corners of the mouth. Those with prolonged iron deficiency also develop brittle and spoon-shaped fingernails.

Iron loss can usually be treated with a balanced diet consisting of a variety of whole foods. Certain foods can decrease the absorption of iron. Grains, certain beans, peanuts, tea, coffee and fermented soy all contain phytates, which are plant compounds that block the absorption of iron. My last point about iron is the use of iron supplements. Taking them if they are not needed can lead to oxidative stress and, for many, constipation.

Clinical Note

Physicians are quick to recommend an iron supplement when someone feels fatigued or tired. Yet an iron supplement should be given only when there is evidence of iron deficiency found in blood work. This will be seen as a low MCV and low MCHC. Other indications of iron deficiency anemia include decreased hematocrit, hemoglobin, and ferritin levels.

Magnesium

Magnesium is needed for many biochemical reactions in the body. It helps to maintain and relax muscles and nerves, supports the immune system, and keeps bones strong. It is needed to produce energy from the foods we eat, to help regulate blood sugar, to promote normal blood pressure, and to help keep the heart rhythm steady. Magnesium also can act as a mild sedative, which allows for a good night's sleep.

Like other minerals, the main reason for magnesium deficiency is a nutrient-deprived diet. Yet gastrointestinal disorders such as Crohn's disease can limit the ability to absorb magnesium, and conditions that create chronic diarrhea can also result in a magnesium deficiency.

This may come as a shock, but alcohol—yes, alcohol—can deplete magnesium. According to the *Journal of the American College of Nutrition,* alcohol consumption acts as a magnesium diuretic, causing a "vigorous" increase in magnesium loss through the urine. Chronic intake of alcohol also depletes the stores of magnesium from the body and decreases its absorption. Alcohol, or ethanol, contributes to vitamin-D deficiency, which can also lower magnesium levels. Chemotherapy, diuretics, antibiotics, physical stress, and excessive exercising also can cause a loss of magnesium.

When magnesium levels get low enough, symptoms occur. You may have heard of cardiac arrhythmias, muscle cramping, and Restless Leg Syndrome. How about anxiety, hyperactivity, and difficulty falling asleep? Adequate magnesium is needed for the brain and nervous system. It is also needed for electrolyte balance, which affects the nervous system.

Ron G. came to me complaining of Restless Leg Syndrome—a set of symptoms characterized by uncomfortable sensations in the legs and an urgency to move the legs. The symptoms always occur at night while resting or trying to sleep. I quickly learned that he enjoyed alcohol at night, and was consuming too many nutrient-deprived foods. Following an assessment of his blood work, along with bioelectrical-impedance testing to evaluate his body fat and metabolism, a food plan was implemented. To help him with the restless legs, I prescribed magnesium glycinate to be taken a few hours before bed. Ron also agreed to reduce his drinking at night. Within a few days the symptoms in his legs disappeared, and he reported sleeping better than he could remember.

Clinical Note

Often I prescribe magnesium once I fully understand a patient's condition and any medications he or she may be taking. When considering whether you should supplement with magnesium or any other nutrient, it's important to know what condition or health issue you are trying to resolve and to determine if those nutrients will be of benefit. Second, there are endless possibilities for interactions between prescription drugs and natural nutrients. Before you take concentrated single nutrients, or supplements with multiple nutrient ingredients, I suggest you consult with a healthcare professional seasoned in nutrition and nutritional biochemistry, to make sure you are not causing any adverse drug-and-nutrient interactions.

Magnesium-rich foods include: almonds, artichoke, avocado, bananas, beans, beef, beets, blackberries, Brazil nuts, butternut squash, cashews, fish, hazelnuts, kiwi, peas, pecans, pistachios, pumpkin seeds, quinoa, raspberries, shrimp, spinach, spirulina, walnuts, and wheat germ.

Manganese

Manganese is needed for enzyme reactions controlling metabolism, energy, and thyroid-hormone function. It is also important in the regulation of blood sugar when we are not eating. A deficiency of manganese is rare. It is abundant in anchovies, asparagus, avocado, bananas, beans, blackberries, blueberries, cranberries, eggs, grapefruit, herring, kale, nuts, pineapple, raspberries, brown rice, sardines, spirulina, squash, strawberries, sweet potatoes, and Swiss chard.

Phosphorous

After calcium, phosphorous is the second most abundant mineral in the body. The skeleton contains roughly 85 percent of total body phosphorous. Besides its role in the structural component of teeth and bones, it is important in maintaining healthy cell membranes, as well as high-energy compounds that are needed for metabolism.

Phosphorous is abundant in many foods, and is well absorbed; therefore, deficiency is highly unlikely. However, those at risk for deficiency are alcoholics and those who abuse antacids containing magnesium and aluminum, which can cause phosphorous malabsorption and increased urinary loss of phosphorous.

Phosphorous is found in artichoke, avocado, most beans, black currants, Brussels sprouts, eggs, fish, kiwi, meat, nuts (including Brazil nuts and cashews), parsnips, peas, poultry, pumpkin seeds, sunflower seeds, and sweet potato.

Potassium

Potassium is the third most abundant mineral in the body. It is needed for nerve firing, muscle contraction, and, more important, proper heart function. Potassium interacts with sodium and chloride to control fluids, pH, and electrolyte balance.

Clinically, I see many endurance athletes who succumb to a loss of potassium, or hypokalemia, due to excessive sweating. They commonly complain of muscle cramping, heart irregularities, fatigue, and weakness. This is due not only to direct loss of potassium, but also to depletion of potassium from the muscles. Potassium is stored with muscle sugar (glycogen), and it is lost when muscles use up the glycogen to get through a workout.

High levels of stress hormones, diuretic use, and malnutrition can also cause hypokalemia. When potassium is deficient, it results in heart failure, muscle weakness, paralysis (in extreme situations), kidney dysfunction, and problems with elevated blood sugar.

If you exercise daily, you should drink water not only all day, but during and right after exercising in order to replenish electrolytes lost in the workout. In the *Rebuild Logbook*, the companion to this book, I have included a tasty, homemade electrolyte recipe to create your own sports drink. I suggest you use it to replenish fluids and electrolytes without wasting money on crappy sports drinks loaded with high-fructose corn syrup.

Potassium-rich foods include almonds, avocado, bamboo shoots, bananas, most beans, beef, bok choy, Brussels sprouts, carrots, cherries, chicken, clams, coconut, dates, fish (especially salmon), grapefruit, kiwi, steel-cut oats, papaya, parsnips, pumpkin seeds, sardines, spinach, sunflower seeds, sweet potatoes, Swiss chard, tomatoes, and turkey.

Selenium

Selenium has two important functions. It is needed to produce a powerful antioxidant that has the ability to render free radicals harmless. More important, it gobbles up the free radicals that damage LDL. Also, due to its role in regulating thyroid hormones, selenium is needed for normal growth and metabolism.

The major food sources of selenium are seafood and organ meats. Other sources include eggs, grains, meat, and poultry. Additional amounts are found in asparagus, bananas, beans, Brazil nuts (highest selenium content), Brussels sprouts, cashews, coconut, parsnips, black-eyed peas, long-grain brown rice, and spinach.

Z Note

The thyroid gland releases small amounts of the hormones T4 and T3. T4 is inactive whereas T3 is active—it drives your metabolism. When iodine is removed from T4, it becomes T3. The removal of iodine from T4 is dependent on selenium.

Sodium

Sodium has gotten a bad rep. In small amounts, sodium is an essential mineral needed to balance fluids and electrolytes, and regulate blood volume and pH. Along with potassium, sodium is needed to transmit nerve impulses and regulate muscle function. However, as we know, Americans eat far too much sodium chloride (salt).

As a daily requirement, the magic number for salt is 2,400 mg, roughly one teaspoon. The American Heart Association recommends no more than 1,500 mg of sodium per day. The concern is that high amounts of dietary salt can lead to increased blood volume and high blood pressure, which can cause heart disease.

If you are salt-sensitive, lowering your intake involves more than just leaving the salt shaker in the spice rack. Unless you are paying attention to food labels or eating mostly home-cooked meals, you are probably getting too much salt in your diet. Most of the salt we get is from processed and fast foods. Let's look at the sodium content of some popular items. For instance, the Big Mac has a "whopping" 970 mg of sodium. McDonald's double cheeseburger has 1,050 mg, and the Premium Crispy Chicken Club Sandwich tops the list at 1,410 mg.

Now let's take a look at popular deli meats. A two-ounce serving (four thin slices) of deli-style smoked ham has about 660 mg of sodium; two ounces of regular ham has 590 mg, and four thin slices of deli turkey breast has 600 mg. While we're on the topic of lunch, let's look at the sodium content of a popular packaged "food-like" product fed to children— Lunchables. Manufactured by Oscar Mayer, the plastic-wrapped turkey-and-cheddar Lunchable contains 1,100 mg of sodium per serving. The recommended daily allowance of sodium for children four to eight years old is 1,200 mg. Don't even get me started on hot dogs—a plain hot dog on a white-flour bun contains 717 mg of sodium; add chili and cheese and you reach 1,264 mg.

What better way to spend a rainy Saturday afternoon than at the movies with a bag of popcorn? Yet movie popcorn is a wolf in sheep's clothing. A large bag of popcorn has 1,500 mg of sodium—and that doesn't include the yellow, buttery stuff they squirt all over it. This "buttery" substance adds nine grams of saturated fat.

Hidden sodium is also found in cured meats (sausage, bacon, and deli meats), breads and other baked goods, microwaveable foods, and many foods from Chinese restaurants. Sodium is added in various forms, such as sodium nitrite, sodium saccharin, sodium benzoate, and monosodium glutamate (MSG, or free glutamic acid).

Most fruits and vegetables are low in sodium; celery is the notable exception. Beef, coconut, eggs, fish, pumpkin seeds, quinoa, and turkey also contain sodium.

Z Note

MSG is a white powder made from the amino acid glutamate, which is found in seaweed, sugar beets, other vegetables, and cereal gluten. The sodium component of MSG turns it into a salt. MSG enhances the flavors of food, and it is added to canned vegetables and soup, processed meats, Chinese food, dressings, junk-food snacks (Doritos, Cheetos, and any snacks with cheese powder), hot dogs, smoked meats, grated parmesan cheese, and soy sauce. MSG is also found in powdered spice packets, soup packets, and dry dressing mix.

Even though it is used in many foods, it can cause many side effects, including migraine headaches, asthma, rashes, hives, vomiting, heart irregularities, depression, flushing, numbness and tingling, nausea, and weakness. To figure out why, I picked up a book called *Excitotoxins: The Taste That Kills,* by Dr. Russell L. Blaylock. He explores the dangers of artificial flavor enhancers like MSG, as well as sweeteners like aspartame. Citing hundreds of scientific studies, Dr. Blaylock has uncovered the harmful effects of MSG on the brain and nervous system.

Basically, glutamate is a naturally occurring amino acid, and its role is to stimulate the brain and nervous system as a neurotransmitter. Under normal levels, it is important for memory, learning, and muscle tone. However, an excess of glutamate can overstimulate the nervous system, causing nerve cell death. MSG is known as an excitotoxin due to its potential role in damaging the nervous system.

If monosodium glutamate can potentially damage the nervous system, can it affect body composition? A study published in the journal *Obesity* linked monosodium glutamate to overweight and obesity. Over 750 Chinese men and women, ages 40 to 59, were studied. Of those who cooked at home, roughly 82 percent used MSG in their food. That group was further divided into three groups. Adjusted for calorie intake and physical activity, those who used the most MSG were three times more likely to be overweight. The study mentioned that MSG can damage appetite control in the brain, as well as affect how we metabolize, or burn, fat.

Zinc

This metallic ion is important in many key functions ranging from carbohydrate-and-protein metabolism, alcohol detoxification, wound healing, vision, growth, balancing blood sugar, smell and taste perception, DNA repair, immune function, and defense against free radicals.

Zinc is important during pregnancy for the growth and development of the fetus, due to the rapid division of cells. Zinc is also needed for growth in infants, children, and teens, and it can help to alleviate symptoms of premenstrual syndrome.

The immune system is dependent on zinc. T lymphocytes are white blood cells that are divided into three types: T cells, B cells, and natural-killer cells. T cells help other white blood cells coordinate the immune response and destroy cells infected by viruses and cancer. B cells are those that make antibodies, which seek and destroy bacteria and viruses. Natural-killer cells are a type of aggressive lymphocyte that also kill cells infected with viruses, as well as cancer cells. When zinc is deficient, these lymphocytes are less able to fight off infection and tumor cells.

Zinc plays a vital role in male and female fertility. It is needed to maintain sperm count, motility, prostate health, and testosterone levels. A study found in the *Asian Journal of Andrology* found zinc levels to be directly related to sperm development and sperm count. A deficiency of zinc was also found to cause a dysfunction of the gonads, as well as testosterone levels.

Zinc-rich foods include: asparagus, avocado, most beans, beef, blackberries, Brussels sprouts, cashews, chicken, eggs, fish, oats, peas, pomegranate, pumpkin seeds, raspberries, brown rice, seafood (especially oysters), spirulina, sunflower seeds, Swiss chard, turkey, and wheat germ.

Rainbow-Colored Disease Fighters

Fruits and vegetables are the most nutrient-dense foods you can eat. They are high in water content and low in calories.

Fruits and vegetables are high in fiber, which satisfies the appetite and improves blood sugar and bowel health. In addition to an abundance of vitamins and minerals, fruits and vegetables contain colored pigments, which are powerful antioxidants that neutralize free radicals formed in the body. A free radical is a simple molecule with a missing electron. To become whole again, free radicals interact with, and steal, electrons from other cells or tissues in the body. Doing so leaves those cells or tissues damaged. This process is called oxidation, which has been linked to many chronic diseases.

In addition to these brilliantly colorful pigments which act as antioxidants, plants contain special phytochemicals (plant chemicals) that can protect against or prevent diseases. Some phytochemicals give fruits and vegetables color, while others provide distinctive tastes and smells. You may be familiar with lycopene, which is found in deep-red tomatoes, or the anthocyanins that create the dark-purple color of blueberries. A compound called allicin, which contains sulphur, is responsible for the smell of garlic, just as catechins in tea cause its slightly bitter taste.

Scientific research shows how these phytochemicals work synergistically with vitamins, minerals, and fiber to provide us with protection from disease. Thousands of plant compounds protect plants in their environment and, when eaten, protect us from disease. As you read, you will discover the major impact they have on the mechanisms of disease.

Red Fruits and Vegetables

The phytochemicals found in red fruits and vegetables comprise a group of valuable compounds: quercetin, ellagic acid, hesperidin, lycopene, and anthocyanins. Lycopene and anthocyanins are powerful antioxidants that provide the red pigments. These nutrients reduce the risk of cancer, reduce tumor growth, lower blood pressure, scavenge free radicals, reduce low-density lipoprotein (LDL), and reduce inflammation in those with arthritis. For that reason, tomatoes are not just tasty; they contain lycopene, which helps to prevent atherosclerosis and coronary-artery disease.

In fact, data found in the *American Journal of Clinical Nutrition* showed lycopene protecting LDL from oxidative stress—a component in the development of coronary-artery disease. The study also found that those with low blood-serum concentrations of lycopene had thicker coronary arteries, a condition associated with atherosclerosis and coronary-artery disease.

The phytochemical quercitin inhibits the growth of colon cancer. A study published in the *International Journal of Cancer* showed that using a very small amount of quercetin, colon-cancer cell growth was halted. According to *Cancer Research*, quercetin was also effective in causing apoptosis (self-initiated cell death) in leukemia and lymphoma cell lines.

The anthocyanins in fruits and vegetables also help to prevent hardening of the arteries, lower blood pressure, reduce inflammation, and prevent cancer. Ellagic acid helps to prevent cancer by neutralizing toxins found in processed meat and tobacco smoke. All of these compounds are found in red apples, beets, cherries, currants, red grapes, guava, kidney beans, red onion, red peppers, radicchio, radishes, raspberries, rhubarb, strawberries, tomatoes, and watermelon.

Blue and Purple Fruits and Vegetables

These have the highest antioxidant action of all plant-based foods, providing anthocyanins, ellagic acid, resveratrol, flavonoids, quercetin, lutein, tannins, and zeaxanthin. Similar to the nutrients in red plant foods, these nutrients lower LDL, improve immune function, support digestion, improve mineral absorption, reduce inflammation, reduce tumor growth, and reduce coronary-artery disease.

Anthocyanin-rich berries are pretty powerful. During the past few decades, research has been done showing the therapeutic effects of anthocyanins on diseases, including cancer. A study was done using an extract made up of six berries—wild blueberry, bilberry, cranberry, elderberry, raspberry, and strawberry—to determine their antioxidant efficacy and anti-angiogenic properties. Angiogenesis is a process whereby cancer cells create blood vessels to supply tumors with blood and nutrients. The six-berry extract was found to inhibit the process of angiogenesis in tumors.

Additionally, anthocyanins protect cells from oxidative stress, improve memory, and lower risk for developing cancer. The plant compounds found in blue/purple/black fruits and vegetables are abundant in black beans, blackberries, black currants, blueberries, purple cabbage, eggplant, elderberries, figs, purple grapes, plums, purple potatoes, prunes, and raisins.

Z Note

Research continues on the health benefits of anthocyanins against chronic disease. Many studies are coming to the same conclusion regarding the effect of anthocyanins found in dark-blue and purple fruits and berries on the mechanisms involved in the development of cardiovascular disease. Two such studies are worth mentioning here. Nitric oxide (NO) is a signaling molecule produced by the single layer of cells (the endothelium) that lines arteries. NO relaxes the muscle within the artery, causing dilation of the arteries, improved blood flow, and reduced blood pressure. Collective data published in *Advances in Nutrition* revealed that anthocyanins found in berries improve the release of nitric oxide and protect the endothelium from damage. It was also noted that anthocyanins shut down the inflammation that is responsible for the development of coronary-artery disease.

In another study published in the journal *Angiology*, researchers found that anthocyanins contained in the nutritional supplement OPC-3 improved circulation and reduced cardiovascular risk factors. A randomized, double-blind, placebo-controlled, parallel group study was conducted. The control group received a two-month supply of OPC-3, which contains extracts from grape seed, bilberry, citrus, pine bark, and red wine. The placebo group received a mixture of fructose, apple fiber, and food dyes. The study showed that those who took the OPC-3 had an improvement in blood pressure and, more impressive, a significant decrease in the inflammatory marker CRP—C-reactive protein. CRP is a major predictor of cardiovascular-disease risk.

Orange and Yellow Fruits and Vegetables

Orange and yellow plant-based foods contain beta-carotene, flavonoids, lycopene, zeaxanthin, and lutein. Beta-carotene is a strong antioxidant that can be converted into vitamin A. It also helps to protect the skin, maintain the immune system, and reduce the risk of blindness and strokes.

Along with protecting your skin and eyes, beta-carotene and lycopene greatly reduce the risk for cancer and heart disease, while lutein and zeaxanthin reduce the risk of disorders of the eye. As reported in *Archives of Ophthalmology*, demographic, lifestyle, and medical characteristics were measured for 4,519 participants aged 60 to 80 years of age. Those with a high dietary intake of lutein and zeaxanthin were less likely to develop age-related macular degeneration of the eyes.

Due to the powerful properties of these phytochemicals, research shows that these carotenoids can also help to detoxify drugs and foreign chemicals. In addition, omitting carotenoid-rich vegetables from your diet may weaken your immune system.

Orange and yellow foods include apricots, butternut squash, cantaloupe, carrots, grapefruit, pumpkins, lemon, mango, nectarines, orange, peaches, pineapple, yellow peppers, orange peppers, peaches, winter squash, sweet potatoes, and tangerines.

Green Fruits and Vegetables

Green leafy vegetables are an excellent source of folate (a B vitamin), potassium, vitamin K, vitamin C, and omega-3 fatty acids. Green vegetables get their different shades of color from a phytochemical called chlorophyll. In addition to chlorophyll, green foods—specifically cruciferous vegetables—contain a class of compounds called organosulfides.

Crucifers such as broccoli, Brussels sprouts, cabbage, cauliflower, and kale are believed to help prevent macular degeneration of the eyes and the formation of cataracts. More important is the protection they provide against cancer. Breast cancer is the most common cancer in women in the United States, and the second leading cause of cancer-related deaths among women. Present treatments include toxic chemotherapy, estrogen modifiers, radiation, and radical mastectomies. However, Mother Nature, in her infinite wisdom, created compounds in the foods we eat to provide protection from breast cells growing out of control. There is now evidence showing that the compounds found in cruciferous vegetables stop the growth of breast cancer. Crucifers accomplish this by making estrogen less potent.

Estrogen is the primary female sex hormone needed for the development of the breasts and maturation of the reproductive system. Once made, estrogen is broken down into two different forms: 2-hydroxy estrogen and 16-hydroxy estrogen. The former prevents breast cells from growing, while the latter causes breast cells to grow.

A chemical known as indole-3-carbinol (I-3-C), found in cruciferous vegetables, can alter estrogen metabolism that can protect women from breast cancer. Studies published in *Cancer Research* and the *Journal of Biological Chemistry* found that I-3-C suppressed the growth of estrogen-dependent and estrogen-independent breast-cancer cell lines by favoring 2-hydroxy estrogen. It was also found that I-3-C shut down breast cancer tumor growth and the spread of breast cancer by deactivating 16-hydroxy estrogen.

It is becoming well known in the scientific community that an unhealthful environment creates the majority of cancers. From BPAs found in most plastics, and the widespread consumption of cow milk, to the standard American diet consisting of nutrient-deficient, high-calorie, processed foods, these unhealthful lifestyle choices seem to be the culprits in triggering the onset and return of cancer.

The good news is that crucifers are also strong detoxifiers, combating and neutralizing cancer-causing agents (carcinogens). These powerful vegetables help clear toxic compounds from the body, whether the compounds come from junk food or the environment.

Carcinogenesis and Crucifers

Normal Cell

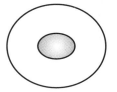

Inflammation, toxins, processed foods, hormones, and free radicals can interrupt and damage the cell's DNA

Phytochemicals protect the cells from DNA damage

Damaged DNA

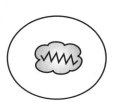

Phytochemicals stop the replication of cancerous cells

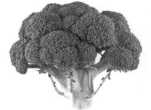

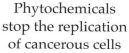

Precancerous Tumor

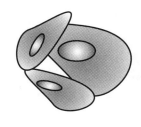

Phytochemicals stop the spread of cancer cells and block the production of blood vessels

Once cancerous cells develop into a tumor, they grow their own blood supply

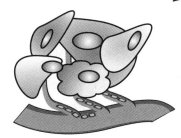

Tumor with blood supply

Green choices include green apples, artichokes, arugula, asparagus, avocados, bok choy, broccoli, Brussels sprouts, green cabbage, celery, chives, cucumbers, herbs, grapes, green peppers, leafy greens, honeydew melon, kale, kiwi, leeks, lettuce, limes, parsley, peas, spinach, Swiss chard, and zucchini.

As I read through the research regarding chronic disease like cancer, heart disease, and Alzheimer's disease, it frustrates me to know that this information is not common knowledge. After all, isn't presenting information and providing tools to prevent disease the purpose of the institutions that raise money to find cures for these chronic illnesses?

White and Tan Fruits and Vegetables

White fruits and vegetables are colored by the pigment called anthoxanthins. They also contain important phytochemicals, such as allicin (found in garlic), organosulfur compounds, fructan, flavonoids, quercetin (found in onions), and beta-glucans (found in mushrooms). These nutrients also stimulate the immune system and reduce the risk of certain cancers.

Cooking is one of those must-do activities to ensure you are getting healthful nutrition. I really enjoy preparing foods when they are in season. During spring and summer, nothing beats dark-green salads with bright and colorful vegetables mixed throughout, and fresh, sweet fruit. During the cool autumn days and the cold winter nights, there is something comforting about hot soups and stews. Regardless of the time of year, there is nothing like the smell of sautéing garlic or onion permeating the house.

Garlic and onion belong to the allium genus of vegetables, which also includes leeks, chives, shallots, and scallions. Besides warding off vampires, garlic has been used for centuries to flavor meals and has been used as medicine all over the world. Garlic has a mixture of phytochemicals, and it also supplies vitamins C and B6. The sulphur compounds in garlic not only provide for its distinctive smell, they are thought to protect against heart disease and cancer. In addition, garlic contains saponins, which add the bitter taste. Saponins have been shown to provide anti-inflammatory and antimicrobial activity against bacteria, yeast, parasites, fungi, and viruses.

Have you ever wondered why you cry when chopping onions? When you cut the flesh of an onion, enzymes are released which then produce sulfenic (not sulphuric) acids. These acids are responsible for forming your tears. Onions also contain sulphur compounds, saponins, fructans, and two major flavonoids: quercetin and kaempferol. Both are powerful antioxidants and are important for immune function and healthy gene expression. Fructans are indigestible parts of the onion, which help to maintain beneficial bacteria in the gut.

What about ginger? Ginger is the root of a plant known for its spicy and sharp taste, as well as its medicinal properties. Its most common use is to soothe the stomach. From acid reflux to motion sickness, the phenols and oils found in ginger can relieve symptoms of the stomach. The nutrients found in this white root can provide pain relief from arthritis, muscle soreness, and menstrual cramps.

Did I forget to mention mushrooms? Mushrooms, such as ganoderma, maitake, shiitake, and white button, are among the many functional foods known to inhibit tumor growth by enhancing immune function. A clinical study reported that beta-glucans—long carbohydrates found in mushrooms— stimulate the cancer-killing white blood cells called natural killer cells. How long did the killing response last? They found the activity of the natural killer cells in lung, breast, and liver cancer to exceed one year. That is *amazing*.

The phytochemicals found in white button mushrooms were also found to inhibit the growth of breast-cancer cells by blocking an enzyme needed for the cellular growth. In addition to these powerhouse phytochemicals, mushrooms are also an excellent source of non-heme iron, phosphorus, potassium, B vitamins, copper, and zinc. In addition, mushrooms provide immunotherapy for anyone with a compromised immune system and those with cancer, especially hormone-sensitive cancers.

Warning: Anyone with known autoimmune disorders may want to steer clear of mushrooms and supplements containing mushroom extracts because of their immune-enhancing activity.

Z Note

Breast-cancer cells produce an enzyme called aromatase, which increases the amount of circulating estrogen by converting other hormones into estrogen. By increasing levels of estrogen, cancer cells can continue to proliferate and spread. Yet a study done by Grube *et al.* found in the *Journal of Nutrition*, showed the phytochemicals in white button mushrooms blocked the production of the aromatase enzyme, which decreased cancer-cell growth. It was also found that the extract from white button mushrooms had no toxic effects.

White fruits and vegetables include bananas, cauliflower, chickpeas, cucumbers, figs, garlic, ginger, great northern beans, Jerusalem artichoke, leeks, lentils, mushrooms, onions, parsnips, pinto beans, shallots, turnips, white corn, white peaches, and white potatoes.

The benefits of nutrients found in plant-based foods goes far beyond a healthy body composition, one that is low-fat and lean. As you can see, fruits and vegetables are among the most nutritious foods that you can eat. They are packed with vitamins, minerals, antioxidants, phytochemicals, and other unique compounds that promote optimal health. By eating a variety of fruits and vegetables of different colors, you are guaranteed a diverse amount of plant-based nutrients needed for optimal health. If you are rebuilding from a health crisis, taking steps to prevent recurrence, prevent chronic disease, and get lean, I recommend five to six servings of vegetables and low-sugar fruits a day. When designing your diet, make sure to include plenty of vegetables and fruits in your meals and certainly when you snack.

Three "Z Rules" for a Healthy Body Composition

Now that we understand more about what foods do inside the body, I'll show you my diet rules. I do not want to provide a complicated regimen for those seeking to change the way they eat. Rules are made to be broken, and that's especially true with people who have tried a dozen different diets and found none of them work. In this book I'm going to keep it simple. I think there are three main reasons for being over-fat. First, people eat high-calorie, nutrient-absent, crappy food. Second, they eat their biggest meal at night. Third, they are not performing the right fat-burning exercises. So I have three rules. That's right, count them. Yet these guidelines will make all the difference in your body composition.

Here are the Z Rules:
1. Eat high-nutrient, low-calorie foods throughout the day (roughly five to six times a day).
2. Eat little to no carbs (especially refined, white carbs), nor a big protein meal, after 6–7 p.m.
3. Burst to burn and rebuild: High-intensity interval training creates a health body composition.

That's not so hard, is it? You don't have to count calories; I've already done it for you. You don't have to cut back on the amount of food you're eating. The tools in this plan will help you eat according to the way your body works best. That's what really cuts down the weight. Let's look at the first rule and see exactly what that means for you.

Z Rule #1. Eat a lot of nutrient-dense foods, and eliminate empty-calorie foods.

OK, how bad is processed, empty-calorie food for you? Let me count the ways. Do you suffer from heart disease, cancer, diabetes, obesity, autoimmune diseases, digestive issues, mood disorders, fatigue, insomnia, sleep apnea, poor healing, hormone imbalances, low libido, skin issues, or arthritis? Are you afflicted with dementia, Alzheimer's disease, ADHD, osteoporosis, immune suppression, or chronic colds and allergies?

You must be suffering from **PFD**—Processed-Food Disorder. This is a condition caused by eating too many highly processed, refined, high-calorie, low-nutrient foods. Why does what you eat matter so much? Research is showing that the chemical composition of these refined grains, sugars, dairy, processed foods, and fast foods talks to genes in a way that causes cells, tissues, and organs to become diseased. Compare that to the information that comes from nutrient-dense, low-calorie whole foods. That turns on a different set of genes that cause the body to work in a normal and healthy way.

You may remember the war the government waged against Big Tobacco in the name of health for American citizens. That same process is going on today—only with the food we can buy at any supermarket in the land. As a person who understands nutrition so well, I am discouraged that the processed and junk-food industry is given a free pass to manufacture, advertise, and distribute synthetic non-foods. More and more, clinical studies are showing that these foods are the source for most, if not all, of our chronic diseases, from diabetes to heart disease to cancer. Meanwhile, small farms producing whole foods are unable to compete in a market where the cost to run the farms is more than the money they can earn. Huge agribusinesses like Monsanto and Perdue use their power in the market and their huge profits to ensure their top position, squashing the small farmers. If we continue to buy processed foods, we are handing over billions of dollars to an industry which could not care less about us.

That's why restricting how many calories you eat is a doomed strategy. The real question is: what are you eating? According to the journal *Nutrition & Metabolism*, restricting calories alone (without exercise) is not a sustainable long-term solution for improving body composition. More than half of the people who lose weight (fat) as a result of restricting calories will regain it. In contrast, researchers have found that a diet high in nutrients and low in calories, with lower carbs, higher protein, and some fat, showed improvements in a lower body-fat percentage and in lean muscle mass—a better body composition.

Dr. Z's Fast Food

Protein

- Rotisserie chicken (hot for one meal, cold for chicken salad)
- Applegate Farms deli meats (turkey, chicken)
- Applegate Farms chicken and turkey sausages (only those with no sugar added)
- Canned tuna (American Tuna brand is low in mercury)
- Sautéed ground meats and vegetables for a quick stew
- Grilled chicken, kebabs, burgers
- Omelets with mushrooms, vegetables

Produce

- Salad mixes, romaine hearts, lettuce, spinach
- Baby carrots (peeled), celery sticks, broccoli florets in bags
- Trader Joe's steamed beets (serve hot, or cold in salads)
- Frozen vegetables and fruits are often as good as fresh, since they are frozen shortly after picking. Peas, lima beans, green beans, edamame, spinach, and berries are available almost everywhere.

Lentils and Grains

- Trader Joe's cooked lentils and rice (basmati, jasmine)
- Eden Organics canned beans (cans are BPA-free)
- Steel-cut oats (cook in quantity and freeze for use later)

Snacks (foods to pack in a cooler and bring to work)

- Nuts (raw walnuts, almonds, peanuts, cashews)
- Seeds (pumpkin, sunflower)
- Nut butters (unsweetened)
- Brown-rice crackers (with nut butter, hummus, avocado)
- Celery or cucumber with nut butter
- Cut carrots, broccoli, cauliflower, apples, sugar-snap peas
- Hummus
- Hard-boiled eggs
- Berries (especially strawberries and blueberries)
- Healthful low-sugar protein bars. Be careful on this one. Many protein bars are very high in sugar. With even low-sugar bars, eat half, then the other half later.

That's because major calorie restriction also means nutrient restriction. A three-year study of the dietary habits of 16,000 Americans found that many people are deficient in nutrients such as vitamin B6, folate, and thiamin, as well as calcium and magnesium. In a scientific review from the *Journal of the American Medical Association,* researchers found that "inadequate intake of several vitamins has been linked to chronic diseases, including coronary-artery disease, cancer, and osteoporosis." The specific vitamins they are referring to are vitamins B6, B12, and folate, as well as vitamins A, C, D, E, and K. If you are eating highly processed foods, or you are severely restricting your calories, you are putting yourself at risk for serious diseases.

Why would trying to lose weight cause these problems? Let's look at the ways your body reacts to the signals you're giving it. By overly restricting calories, your appetite increases and the sense of being full decreases. This not only creates a craving for food, it causes frequent overeating of high-calorie, low-nutrient foods. That happens because the body goes into starvation mode. It doesn't use the fat you have stored up. Instead, it hangs onto fat as an emergency energy source. In starvation mode, the body reacts by breaking down muscle rather than fat. That is an unhealthy cycle that only gets worse.

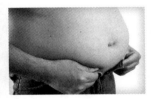
The chronic diseases of Western society—cancer, heart disease, diabetes, high blood pressure, obesity, and arthritis—are directly related to the types of food you eat. Processed and refined foods are usually high in calories and devoid of vital nutrients. These processed foods are not only available and affordable; they are appealing because they taste good and make us feel good in the short term.

Diets that promote severely restricting calories and important food groups deprive you of vital nutrients and calories. By doing so, they can cause you to hold onto fat and cause a slow deterioration of your health. Realize that food is information. When you eat healthful protein, greens, fats, carbs, and other plant-based nutrients, those foods regulate your body functions, cellular functions, and genes. By eating a non-processed, highly nutritious diet, you stop making fat and also prevent and reverse disease. Your fork, not your genes, determines your fate.

If nutrient-dense foods prevent disease and help you get rid of fat, are there foods that can make you ill and increase fat? Let's look at a few food sources that we consume every day—foods that many of us have been eating since childhood. The problem is that scientific evidence is showing that some foods can make us both fat and sick. What those foods are might surprise you. But you know what they say: the truth will set you free—free to make you feel a whole lot better about yourself.

Through years of scientific research, I have learned some alarming facts about three basic food sources in our diet. These are: refined breads and cereal grains; dairy; and refined, processed sugars. That's right, the three worst sources of food are bread, dairy, and sugar—what I call the "Three Foods That Kill." That sounds outrageous, doesn't it? Let's take a closer look, though, at what clinical tests have to show us.

Our Worst Friends

If presented with a choice between an apple and a Snickers bar, or a salad and cheese-covered nachos, we would all acknowledge that the apple and salad are the more healthful food choices. At a restaurant, if I told you that a plate of rice, vegetables, and gooey orange chicken was loaded with monosodium glutamate (MSG, a synthetic salt), most people would think twice before eating it. The point is that we are able to make conscious decisions about the food we choose to eat.

However, there are foods we consume daily that we don't really think about. We don't think they can cause any health issues. We start the day with them, and eat them for lunch and dinner, as though they are the foods we're supposed to be eating. After all, we were brought up with those foods; they are now part of our culture. They are so ingrained in our society that eating "healthy"—the way we were meant to eat—has become the radical view, whereas PFD has become the norm. You will be surprised when I tell you the facts about three of the most popular foods in our kitchens.

Breads/Grains

Before the agricultural revolution (roughly 10,000 years ago), humans were hunter-gatherers. They rarely ate any cereal grains (wheat, maize, rice, barley, sorghum, oats, rye, and millet) because those are produced mostly by farming. Our forebears' food sources consisted of wild meats, fruits, and vegetables. For the last two million years, our genetic makeup was shaped by the food sources that were commonly consumed; cereal grains were not. According to Loren Cordain, Ph.D.,

I Lost 100 Pounds of Fat!

I remember being overweight. I could not go up a flight of stairs without being winded and starting to sweat. I was easily fatigued and suffered from backaches. I felt very tired and sluggish throughout the day. I realized it was time to change my body composition.

To start, I got rid of bread, dairy, and sugar. I got back to the gym and started training four to five days a week. The greatest change I made was not eating after 7 p.m. My diet now consists of eating either eggs with fruit or oatmeal with fruit for breakfast. A few hours later I will have a granola bar with fruit. For lunch I have a turkey wrap and more fruit. I try to snack throughout the day to keep my metabolism high to burn fat. I drink at least a gallon of water throughout the day. My dinner is either steak or chicken, grilled or baked, with a cup of wild rice or salad.

Following the rules in the Body Composition Diet, I went from 293 pounds to 186 pounds. I began dieting and exercising to lose weight and become generally healthier. It was a lifestyle change. I have become ten times more active and much happier now that I have lost so much weight. I do not feel fatigued throughout the day, and my energy level has gone through the roof.

Thank you!

José B.

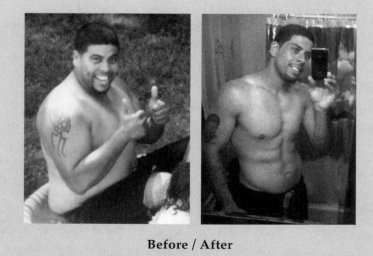

Before / After

in an article titled "Cereal Grains: Humanity's Double-Edged Sword," the addition of cereal grains to our diets roughly 10,000 years ago "represents a dramatic departure from those foods to which we are genetically adapted." He also states that the addition of grains into our modern diet is responsible for many of the current chronic diseases.

To begin with, even before processing, cereal grains do not contain such vital nutrients as vitamin A, beta-carotene, vitamin B12, vitamin C, and vitamin D. In order to make bread, cereal grains have to be processed. The processing causes depletion of the nutrients the grains contain naturally, so breads and flours have to be fortified. The missing nutrients are added in order to create nutritional value. Furthermore, when people eat breads and cereal grains, they tend to eat less meat, fruits, and vegetables. That causes even more nutrient deficiencies.

Consuming breads not only puts us at risk for chronic disease, it also makes us fat. Bread is a carbohydrate. Once eaten, it is broken down into sugars that spike insulin, which starts the cycle for making fat.

Susan Q. came to see me with fatigue, major stomach pain after eating, and aches and pains, as well as a general sense of not feeling well. She also suffered from chronic neck pain. As with most patients I see, I tried to get to the root of her health issues in order to find the most effective treatment. My tentative diagnosis for Susan was that she had either food allergies, an infection in her gut, or a sensitivity to gluten. Because blood testing was the most logical place to start, I had her tested for sensitivity to gluten. The tests came back positive. Because this is a serious issue, I recommended Susan eliminate any grain containing gluten. Those include wheat, barley, rye, refined breads, kamut, spelt, and triticale. Within days, Susan's stomach started to feel better, and her fatigue diminished. Now, more aware and gluten free, she can make food choices that won't be hazardous to her health.

The cereal grains wheat, barley, and rye contain the proteins gluten and gliadin. Gluten is what makes dough pliable and elastic. Because cereal grains are not really meant for human consumption, the gluten in grains can cause an immune reaction in the gut that causes white blood cells to destroy the intestinal lining. This serious condition is called celiac disease. Other autoimmune diseases which have been associated with grain consumption include dermatitis, insulin-dependent diabetes, Hashimoto's thyroiditis, rheumatoid arthritis, nephropathy (kidney disease) and, possibly, multiple sclerosis. In fact, the gluten hazard is now so well known that many gluten-free cookbooks have come out loaded with recipes—gluten-free this and gluten-free that. Researchers and consumers are realizing that many foods contain gluten and, thus, cause health problems. Due to this awareness, food companies are jumping on the gluten-free bandwagon.

Some diets even advocate eating no grains at all. That's too bad, because that overstates the case. There are two types of grains: refined grains and whole grains. Refined grains have been stripped of the bran, germ, and fiber by the process of sifting or grinding. Bran, in its natural state, is the protective outer layer that contains fiber. The germ is the part of the seed that sprouts; it contains vitamins and minerals. The endosperm is the starchy inside that is used to make flour. The ground grain is then bleached and bromated, a process where the chemical bromine is added to assist in making dough stronger. After the chemical change, processed-food companies add B vitamins and iron to the flour in an attempt to restore what has been depleted by the refinement process. Even so, refined flours and grain are still devoid of nutrients and fiber. Examples of refined flours and grains include white flour, white rice, wheat flour, cornmeal, cream of wheat, cream of rice, and most baked goods, such as cookies, pies, cakes, and muffins.

Refined grains are hazardous for several reasons:
* They have no fiber.
* They are too starchy and cause rapid blood-sugar spikes.
* Many chemicals are added to refine grains and bread products.
* They have to be enriched because they are nutritionally naked.

- ✦ Bleaches are used to change the color.
- ✦ Artificial flavorings and colors are added to make them pretty and tasty.

Whole grains, in comparison to refined, still contain the bran, germ, and endosperm. Because whole grains still are in their whole form and have not been destroyed through refinement, it would make sense that eating whole grains is the more healthful choice.

I realize it would be hard to eliminate all grains from your diet. Based on the current research, I recommended no refined flours or grains. OK, perhaps a cookie once in a while, or a piece of birthday cake on *your* birthday. Eating junk once in a while is different than making it a part of your daily or weekly diet. Based on my reading and observations, I find brown rice, buckwheat, steel-cut oats, millet, quinoa, and most foods labeled "whole grain" to be the least problematic. That's because preparation of these grains involves soaking or boiling, which helps to break down phytates and other chemicals that prevent absorption of nutrients. I have included some super-tasty recipes in the back of the book that contain brown rice, quinoa, and steel-cut oats. When you create a custom food plan for yourself, after reading the "Enjoy" chapter, remember to *eat grains sparingly*. However, if you have an auto-immune problem, or you have digestive trouble when eating grains, absolutely stay away from both refined and whole grains containing gluten.

Dairy

It has long been heralded as the ultimate source of calcium for our bones. An advertisement used to say, "It does a body good." We got it in school lunches; we dipped cookies in it, and even added additional sugar and food dyes to create new flavors. It has become a staple in American culture, like Superman. This iconic food source is **milk**.

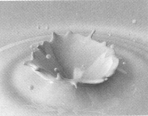

This food has some very good properties. Breast milk is the primary food source for a developing newborn before the introduction of solid foods. In addition to its nutrients, breast milk also contains growth factors, antimicrobials (virus and bacteria fighters), cytokines (signaling molecules that allow communication between cells), and hormones.

Yet the milk we drink is not human breast milk. We drink the milk of another species, and that is abnormal. We are the only mammals who drink milk as adults, and it's not even our own milk. Here are a few reasons why we should not drink milk. Cow milk has roughly three times the amount of protein as human breast milk. The protein component in cow milk is suited for the development of calves, which grow to weigh 1,320 pounds at maturity. I don't know of any 1,300-pound humans. Cow milk also has a higher ratio of casein to whey—typically 80:20. These same two proteins in human milk have a ratio of roughly 40:60. The high proportion of casein in cow milk has been linked to many health issues in humans, specifically allergies and type 1 diabetes.

More and more research is coming to the same conclusion: Milk does a body bad. According to the journals *Medical Hypothesis, The American Journal of Clinical Nutrition,* and *Cancer Epidemiology, Biomarkers & Prevention,* dairy products have been linked to breast cancer, colorectal cancer, and prostate cancer. The American Academy of Pediatrics now recommends that cow milk not be given to an infant during the first year of life. Research is finding that giving infants cow milk may cause the immune system to attack the body, thus creating conditions like type 1 diabetes.

If you still aren't convinced, think about it this way. Did you know cow milk contains white blood cells (pus)? When the udder of a cow is infected by milking machines and human hands, white blood cells rush in to fight the infection. The dairy industry monitors the amount of white blood cells in milk, designated as the "somatic cell count"—a measure of the level of infection in the cows. These white blood cells are passed into the milk that you drink . . . gross!

Brett H., a young businessman, suffered from an inflammatory condition in his colon called colitis. He often had debilitating symptoms of pain, blood in his stool (poop), and fatigue. He was afraid to leave the house, and always had to be near a restroom in case of an emergency. His biggest heartbreak was not being able to sit in a stadium to watch his favorite baseball or football team. General practitioners offered him no solutions, only symptomatic relief. Treatment consisted of steroids and super-strong anti-inflammatories that made him feel tired. After our first consultation, he immediately eliminated grains containing gluten, as well as all dairy products, including milk and cheese. He wasn't a big vegetable eater, but agreed to eat four to five servings of greens a day. To cool the inflammation in his gut, I recommended the powdered amino acid glutamine, a fish-oil supplement, and an anti-inflammatory probiotic. We communicated every couple of weeks to discuss his health and any changes in his colitis. Within two months, Brett returned to my office elated to tell me he had stopped taking the powerful drugs, and had few, if any, symptoms of the colitis. Play ball!

I'd like to share another quick story with you. I was treating a family for a host of physical ailments resulting mainly from physical activity and sports. The youngest son, Sam, was in high school and having a hard time getting through soccer season because of chronic hip and leg pain. After a thorough examination, I found the cause of his hip and leg pain to be a weak hip flexor (psoas). I treated him with manipulation and prescribed home exercises that were to be done daily. In only half a dozen visits, his pain was gone and life was good again. His mother, Lia, pleased with his results, wondered if I could help her younger daughter, Nina, who was struggling with eczema on her arms and legs. I suggested she eliminate dairy from her diet and substitute it with rice milk or almond milk. After several months Lia ecstatically reported that Nina's eczema had cleared up, and Sam was still pain free.

The dairy industry wants us to drink milk and eat cheese because that's their business. In the same way, fast-food companies want us to eat their deep-fried foods, and the tobacco companies would like us to keep smoking—all because they want us to buy their products. Oddly, if I handed you a glass of human breast milk to add to your coffee, I'm sure you'd be grossed out. However, to millions of people, drinking the milk from the udder of a pregnant cow is normal.

Are there any dairy products you can have? No, not even regular ice cream, cheeses, and regular yogurt. Read the previous paragraph again. I know this goes against all we've been told, but it's true. The good news is that the food industry has seized the opportunity and is providing more nutritious and better-tasting substitutes for cow and goat milk. These include rice milk, almond milk, and coconut milk. Rice milk and almond milk are delicious in steel-cut oats, protein shakes, and smoothies. Coconut milk and almond milk are excellent in coffee and make super-delicious ice cream and yogurt. But that doesn't mean you should polish off an entire container of it, like Bruce.

Bruce came to me after being hounded by his daughter to get on a healthful diet to lose weight. Bruce was a hardworking 56-year-old guy who loved to eat. He wanted to lose fat, but he knew nothing about food or how to prepare it, so he ate junk and fast food. He also had an addictive personality and loved ice cream. After learning the consequences of eating poorly, he agreed to eliminate dairy, including ice cream. Once he discovered coconut-milk ice cream, he found it was just as addictive as regular ice cream.

Wait! What about calcium? "We need to drink milk to get calcium for our bones." No, not really. For years the dairy industry has brainwashed us to think we have to drink milk to get calcium. However, current research is showing little evidence to support this propaganda . . . I mean claim. According to the journal *Pediatrics,* Amy Joy Lanou, Ph.D., and Neal Barnard, M.D., reviewed collective studies on dairy consumption, high calcium intake, and bone-mineral density. They found that high calcium intake from milk and dairy products had no impact on bone mineralization in children. Additional research shows that although the United States is one of the highest consumers of dairy products, its rate of osteoporosis and bone fractures is also very high. According to

American Journal of Public Health, in the Nurses' Health Study involving 77,761 women 34 to 59 years old, the women were followed for 12 years. They found that women who consumed dairy products had significantly *more* bone fractures than those who drank little to no milk.

Milk does a body bad. Dark-green vegetables and healthful protein are better sources of calcium.

Sugars—Not So Sweet

We saw earlier in the chapter that different sugars are metabolized differently. Refined sugars (sucrose) and synthetic sugars (high-fructose corn syrup) are very common ingredients in processed foods. Sucrose has different aliases: table sugar, white sugar, and cane sugar. Table sugar is completely devoid of nutrients and loaded with calories. If used in high amounts, sucrose can act as a preservative; therefore, it is found in just about all baked goods, desserts, and junk foods. In other words, you're getting fat so that food-industry products can have a longer shelf life.

High-fructose corn syrup (HFCS) is an industrialized sweetener made from corn, unlike sucrose, which is made from sugar cane and sugar beets. Like sucrose, high-fructose corn syrup has no fiber, which causes the body to process it faster. The consumption of sucrose and high-fructose corn syrup has been proven to help cause heart disease, diabetes, and obesity, among many other serious health issues. These sugars also cause the development of visceral fat (fat surrounding the organs), which for both men and women can cause abnormally high estrogen levels and elevated C-reactive protein, a protein that indicates that your fat has become toxic. Visceral fat also increases your risk for diabetes, heart disease, and certain cancers.

A very useful guide to knowing how your body's sugar levels respond to certain foods is the glycemic index (GI). The GI is an estimate of how much each gram of carbohydrate in a food will raise a person's blood sugar (glucose) after that food is eaten. In this rating system, pure glucose has a value of

100. Carbohydrates that break down quickly during digestion are given a high glycemic index, while carbs that break down more slowly have a low glycemic index.

What is the significance of the glycemic index?

+ Low GI means a smaller rise in blood-glucose levels after meals.
+ Low-GI diets can help you lose weight.
+ Low-GI diets can improve the body's sensitivity to insulin.
+ High-GI foods help to refuel carbohydrate stores after exercise.
+ Low-GI diets can improve control of diabetes.
+ Low-GI foods keep you feeling fuller for longer.
+ Low-GI diets can prolong physical endurance.

Glycemic Index Range

Low GI = 55 or less
Medium GI = 55–69
High GI = 70 or more

If you eat foods with a high glycemic index, you will digest them fast, which will raise your blood sugar fast. High and fast blood sugar means high insulin, and insulin is the hormone that makes you fat.

The higher the number given to a food source, the higher the blood sugar response. For example: watermelon has a glycemic index of 70, which is a high value. Eating watermelon will cause a high blood-sugar response. Peanuts have a low glycemic index of 14, so they don't raise the blood sugar too much or too fast.

As mentioned before, foods that raise blood sugar also raise the hormone insulin. Insulin works by stimulating the cells within your body to take up the glucose in your blood, to be used for energy. The problem with high-glycemic foods is that they cause a quick rise in insulin with a subsequent quick drop in blood sugar. This drop in sugar is known as hypoglycemia, which is the typical crash you get after eating refined carbs and high-sugar foods.

Some foods have a high glycemic index, but they don't have the same blood-sugar response. For example, carrots have a high glycemic index, but don't raise blood sugar like white refined pasta. Why is that? Since we tend to eat only a small amount of carrots, the blood-sugar response is minor. Also, eating foods containing fiber will help to slow the absorption of sugars, preventing a fast rise in blood sugar—unlike white refined flours and sugars, which have no fiber and, thus, cause a rapid rise in blood sugar

If you have a health issue like diabetes or hypoglycemia, or you are trying to lose fat, eat healthful foods and be mindful of the glycemic index. Check the lists of foods provided here and in the next chapter. If you have a problem managing your blood sugar in conditions like insulin resistance or type 2 diabetes, try to stay away from the high-glycemic fruits: banana, mango, papaya, pineapple, and watermelon. This recommendation is not forever, just until you get your blood sugar under control.

Bread, dairy, and sugar are among the foods we eat most, and yet they have the potential to cause a world of health problems. Crazy, right? New patients always say to me, "If I can't eat bread, dairy, or sugar, what do I eat?" I'm sure you are thinking the same thing. Yet you don't need to convert to a new food religion. You just need to stop being a "processed foodatarian," someone who eats packaged foods, fast foods, and foods found in convenience stores and giant warehouses where tires are sold.

You also should avoid a diet that completely cuts out a primary food source, thereby depriving you of vital nutrients. The scientific community is clear on this point. Eating a diet from a variety of food sources is the most healthful way, not just to lose fat, but also to prevent disease.

What do you call someone who eats nutrient-dense, low-calorie, grass-fed meats, organic poultry and eggs, wild seafood (not farm raised), vegetables, fruits, raw nuts and seeds, and healthful fats from avocados and cold-processed oils? I call that person a *varietarian*. I eat a variety of super-healthful whole-food sources, which provide me with all macronutrients (proteins, fats, and carbs), vitamins, minerals, phytochemicals (from plants), and water.

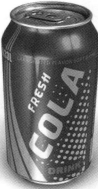

The foods you eat should be nutrient-dense, not calorie-dense. Why don't we look at a common example? Compare a cup of broccoli to a cup of soda. The cup of broccoli has roughly 30 to 40 calories, whereas a cup of soda (cola) has roughly 140 calories. Broccoli has very few calories but is super-high in nutrients. Cola is high-calorie and has absolutely no nutrients. If you drink soda and eat broccoli, you are sending conflicting signals to your body.

Here is another example: One cup of blueberries has roughly 80 calories and is loaded with nutrients, while one cup of Ben and Jerry's Chocolate Chip Cookie Dough ice cream has 540 calories and little to no nutrient value. Blueberries are both high in nutrients and low in calories. Simply by switching from one to the other, you are providing the nutrients that allow your body to work in its most efficient manner.

Alcohol and Nutrient Deficiency

When counseling people on nutrition and exercise, the most common question I hear is, "What about alcohol?" I realize that telling you that you shouldn't drink alcohol creates resistance. However, if you are facing a health issue, I would say give it up. I'm not saying you can't have a drink once in a while. That's your decision. To help you, I will give you the facts on alcohol consumption—then you can decide.

Besides being the number-one recreational drug and the number-one cause of liver cirrhosis, alcohol is one of the main causes of nutrient malabsorption and malnutrition in the United States. Alcohol (ethanol) causes malabsorption of vitamins A, B1, B6, folate, magnesium, potassium, and zinc. It is also a diuretic, causing a loss of water and electrolytes. The health issues that can arise from ethanol include pancreatitis, liver cirrhosis, fatty liver, hemorrhagic stroke, gastrointestinal issues, muscle wasting in the limbs, and an increased risk for cancers of the esophagus, stomach, small intestine, colon, and bladder, as well as estrogen-sensitive breast cancer. Lung cancer is also a major risk because of the synergistic effects of drinking and smoking. Drinking ethanol also increases susceptibility to the painful arthritis, gout.

After ingestion of ethanol, enzymes in the body turn it into acetaldehyde. This compound is more toxic than the alcohol itself. Acetaldehyde can damage the liver, cause free-radical damage, and create the hangover effect. Acetaldehyde is also responsible for causing flushing of the face and a blotchy appearance on the skin, including the reddish/purple tone commonly seen on the nose.

Ethanol also disrupts multiple metabolic pathways in the body that can affect your body composition. It can cause muscle wasting and increased body fat. You may be familiar with a connection between drinking alcohol and unhealthful eating. Sipping on wine or having a cocktail often involves eating cheese and crackers, bread, and/or fried foods. As you become more intoxicated, you start to care less about what and how much you're eating. Both of these scenarios increase your calories and sugars, which causes your body to make fat. Second, having more than one drink introduces more calories than you burn, causing you to store those calories as fat.

Last, drinking ethanol has a dramatic effect on how you burn fat. Inside your body, acetaldehyde is rapidly converted into acetate—a short-chain fatty acid that the body uses for energy. The problem arises because you are burning acetate for energy instead of burning your own body fat.

Warning: Taking acetaminophen (Tylenol) after drinking creates a toxin called NAPQI (pronounced nap-key), which is harmful to the liver.

FOOD SUBSTITUTIONS

Instead of this . . .	Use this . . .
DAIRY from cows, goats, sheep	
Milk	Rice milk, almond milk, coconut milk, or hemp milk
Yogurt	Yogurt made with coconut milk, almond milk, or rice milk
Cream	Coconut-milk creamer (unsweetened) Coconut cream Almond milk thickened with rice flour
Cheese	Daiya™ dairy-free cheese *(see Resources)*
Butter	Grapeseed oil for high-heat cooking; olive oil and others for flavor; avocado *(see OILS & FATS)*
Ice Cream	"Ice cream" made with coconut milk, almond milk, or rice milk
SWEETENERS	
Natural Sweeteners Sugar (cane, brown, raw) Evaporated cane sugar Dextrose Glucose Sucrose Corn syrup High-fructose corn syrup Maple syrup Maltodextrin Sugar alcohols (Erythritol, Maltitol, Mannitol)	In *very* small amounts: Agave nectar Coconut palm sugar Fructose (fresh fruit, dried fruit) Honey (organic only)
Artificial Sweeteners Aspartame (Equal) Saccharine (Sweet'N Low) Sucralose (Splenda)	Rebaudioside or reb A (Rebiana) Stevia (Stevia, Sweet Leaf)

Instead of this . . .	Use this . . .
GRAINS (pasta, bread, and other baked goods)	
Wheat Wheat pasta Rye Barley Oats (rolled, instant) Corn	Brown rice Brown-rice pasta Wild rice Quinoa Oats (steel cut) Almond flour, coconut flour
OILS & FATS	

Hydrogenated and partially
  hydrogenated oils
Corn oil
Soybean oil
Cottonseed oil
Sunflower oil
Processed vegetable oils
Shortening
Lard
Butter
	Grapeseed oil (for high-heat cooking)
	Olive oil (for salads and flavor)
	Avocado oil (for high-heat cooking
	  and flavor)
	Coconut oil (for baking)
	Nut oils (almond, walnut for flavor)

SALT	
Iodized salt	Sea salt Himalayan salt Kosher salt (without additives)
CONDIMENTS	

Ketchup (processed)
Any condiment containing
  sugars, preservatives,
  high-fructose corn syrup,
  or artificial color
	Ketchup (sweetened with agave)
	Tomato paste
	Bragg Liquid Aminos *(see Resources)*
	Umeboshi plum vinegar
	Tamari
	Gluten-free soy sauce

Supplements to Rebuild

Modern agricultural practices and the depletion of nutrients in the soil, coupled with processed nutrient-deprived foods, the onslaught of environmental pollutants, and increasing use of pharmaceuticals, have created a widespread chronic nutrient deprivation. For example, it's a well known fact that cholesterol-lowering drugs cause the depletion of coenzyme Q10—a vitamin-like substance needed to produce energy—while smoking causes a rapid depletion of vitamin C. Sadly, without vital vitamins, minerals, and other plant-based compounds, over time we slowly develop tissue-and-organ dysfunctions and, eventually, chronic disease. Nutritional supplements, such as vitamins, minerals, probiotics, herbs, and enzymes, provide a portion of the daily nutritional needs—filling in the pot holes—for people who could become ill due to lack of proper nutrition to support toxic and stressful lifestyles.

It is well established in the scientific literature that nutraceuticals (supplements) are also important for anyone recovering and rebuilding from disease and/or a medical procedure. For example, in the journal *Cancer Research* the compounds indole-3-carbinol, curcumin, and epigallo-catechin-3-gallate (EGCG, found in green tea) not only prevented cancer, but these dietary compounds in combination with cancer therapies enhanced the antitumor activity of the therapies. The same dietary compounds were also shown to decrease the toxicity caused by chemotherapy and radiation. Regarding heart disease, the *New England Journal of Medicine* found vitamin E to be a powerful antioxidant that prevented the oxidation of LDL—a crucial step in the development of atherosclerosis and coronary-artery disease. Last, *Diabetes Care* and *Diabetology & Metabolic Syndrome* report that zinc and magnesium were found to help reduce the risk of diabetes, as well as to regulate high blood sugar associated with diabetes.

While rebuilding myself from toxic chemotherapy, radiation and surgery, I ate a whole-food diet consisting of plant-based foods, healthful protein, fats and carbs. To supplement that diet, I took probiotics and digestive enzymes, vitamin C, vitamin D, B vitamins, anti-inflammatory nutrients, a multivitamin, essential fats, and specific herbs shown to improve bone-marrow suppression and anemia. I was able to reverse the side effects and recover quickly with my diet and supplement protocol. Taking supplements to recover, rebuild and heal is essential; however, what worked for me may not work for you. As outlined in this book, eating nutrient-dense foods, including plenty of plant-based foods, protein, fats, and healthful carbs based on your *specific* metabolic needs is the most important step in getting rid of fat, and rebuilding yourself from a chronic health issue. *Supplements are not a replacement for a healthful diet.* They are intended to fill in any gaps and add therapeutically to the diet to offset extra stress and facilitate healing and repair.

When considering nutritional support, there are some things you should keep in mind:

* Be aware that some medications and/or medical conditions do not pair well with certain supplements. For example, St. John's Wort (an herbal supplement) should not be taken with antidepressant medication. Consult with a health professional who is well-versed in nutrition to find out if any supplements can affect the intended use of the medication you take, and to make sure there are no contraindications.
* Consider your specific needs. Are you looking for a multivitamin, a specialty product, or help with a specific health condition? Are you currently being treated for a health condition, or rebuilding from one? Medications can cause depletion of some vitamins and minerals, so it's important to know what nutrient(s) may be lost due to a specific drug.
* You should know that certain vitamins work together, *i.e.*, Vitamin C and Vitamin E, when deciding what to take.
* Choose a company that uses good manufacturing practices (GMP), pharmaceutical-grade production and ingredients, and strict quality-control measures.

+ Look for supplements that are tested and analyzed for quality and purity, and have been shown to be effective for their intended use.

There is no one-size-fits-all supplement plan that will work for everyone. However, as part of your program to rebuild, you may want to consider the following:

+ A probiotic to re-inoculate the gut. Pharmaceuticals, including chemotherapy, antibiotics, and steroids, can wipe out normal gut flora. That depletion then contributes to nutrient malabsorption and an overgrowth of unhealthful bacteria along with other problematic organisms.

+ Digestive enzymes taken with each meal will help you break down your food so you can digest and absorb nutrients more efficiently. Enzymes will also help to reduce the inflammation produced by certain foods.

+ Glutamine, deglycyrrhizinated licorice (DGL), and aloe vera are nutrients that support and help to heal the intestinal lining, which supports digestion and immune function. This is very important for anyone with leaky gut syndrome—a condition of compromised gut function where foreign proteins pass through the intestinal lining into the body. Those proteins can cause an immune reaction and inflammation. This is seen in different autoimmune diseases and some cancers.

+ Vitamin D is mandatory for good health. Extensive research has repeatedly shown that a deficiency of vitamin D has been linked to most of the major chronic diseases. Read the section titled "Vitamin D: A Powerful Hormone" starting on page 53.

+ Antioxidants, including vitamin C, vitamin E, beta-carotene, and grapeseed extract, are important for neutralizing free radicals and preventing them from causing damage. Vitamin E and vitamin C are important in protecting LDL from oxidation—a crucial step in the development of atherosclerosis—and preventing DNA damage in cells that can lead to the development of cancer.

- Detoxifying nutrients, such as indole-3-carbinol, selenium, and N-acetylcysteine are all important in improving hepatic (liver) detoxification while reducing inflammation. Indole-3-carbinol is found in cruciferous vegetables. Its benefits are discussed in the section titled "Green Fruits and Vegetables" starting on page 72.
- Omega-3 essential fatty acids. Chemotherapy, specifically the drug vincristine, can cause peripheral neuropathy (tingling) in the hands and feet due to nerve damage. The DHA (docosahexaenoic acid) and EPA (eicosapentaenoic acid), components of fish oil, can assist in healing the damaged nerves. DHA and EPA are also important to reduce inflammation seen in atherosclerosis and other inflammatory diseases.
- A multivitamin/mineral formula will provide an array of vitamins and minerals that can be lost due to pharmaceutical use and/or trauma from surgery. A powdered multivitamin in an isotonic formula is warranted after gastric-bypass surgery, as this type of surgery causes malabsorption and severe nutrient deficiency. Read "Risky Procedures" on page 48.

Note: If you suffer from GERD (gastroesophageal reflux disease, commonly referred to as acid reflux) or an ulcer, you may have a bacterial infection, H. Pylori. The best way to test for that is stool testing. I use and recommend the testing from BioHealth Laboratory (www.biohealthlab.com).

Warning: Whatever you do, stay away from the high-sugar meal-replacement drinks like the classic one given in hospitals to patients with advanced disease – Ensure. Why? An eight-ounce bottle of Ensure has 22 grams of sucrose (table sugar), almost as much as an eight-ounce bottle of Coca Cola, which has 27 grams of sucrose. Sucrose is a major contributor to the development of diabetes, cancer, heart disease, Alzheimer's disease, obesity, and cavities.

Again, nutritional supplements are important for anyone rebuilding from a disease or procedure, or for those wanting to fill in the potholes. Be sure to consult with a qualified health professional, who can assist in developing a plan based on your specific needs.

Time to Indulge

Now that you have a basic understanding of food, let's talk about eating it. In the "Enjoy" chapter I have provided a method to calculate the amount of food you should eat geared specifically to your metabolism. Just like getting a custom suit, dress, or shoes made, the formulas give you a way to find out how much food you require in order to lose fat. The process allows you to create a custom-tailored food plan.

According to nutritional research, each meal should consist of roughly 30 percent protein, 20 percent fat, and 50 percent carbohydrates. This provides you with not only a variety of food sources, but also the nutrients needed to get rid of fat and restore your health. You will notice that, in addition to three meals a day, I have provided three snacks, which allow you to eat foods like fruits, nuts, and seeds. Snack time allows you to eat more calories, as well as additional food sources that provide you with an array of plant-based phytochemicals (plant nutrients). Plant-based foods are loaded with fiber and water, both of which will satisfy your hunger and provide you with nutrients to aid in digestion, regulate hormones, burn fat, and prevent and reverse disease. So, you eat five to six times a day, specifically tailored to the needs of your body . . . period. In the following chapter, I have included an example of a custom meal plan for one day based on two different caloric requirements. You can use something similar, or create your own eating plan based on your individual formula. How cool is that? You can create a custom food plan that's suited just to you.

Dr. Z's Indulging Tips and Tools

1. Whatever you do, don't skip breakfast. According to the *American Journal of Clinical Nutrition*, skipping breakfast can make you fat. Skipping breakfast alters the way insulin talks to the cells. This increases blood sugar, which is then stored as fat. So, start the day with protein and a complex carb. Check out the breakfast ideas in the recipe section.

2. Remember to eat frequently, five or six times a day. This allows better blood-sugar control, increases your metabolism, feeds the muscles, and gets rid of the fat.

3. Spice it up. Adding healthful spices to pop the flavors of food makes eating enjoyable and tasty. Examples of healthful spices include: curry, mustard, ginger, oregano, basil, parsley, cayenne pepper, cumin, and garlic. In this chapter, I have included a long list of spices that go well with specific foods, including poultry, beef, fish, eggs, vegetables, soups, and stews.

4. Drink six to eight glasses of water per day. Water transports oxygen and nutrients to the cells, detoxifies them, helps to regulate body temperature, boosts metabolism, and moisturizes joints, as well as a thousand other benefits. Most of us are "dry"—walking around dehydrated. We lose water constantly throughout the day, especially during the warmer months due to sweating. You can't replace it by downing coffee or a beer. Alcoholic and caffeinated drinks are diuretics, which cause you to lose water. In the journal *Metabolism,* researchers found that hydrating the body increases fat burning. In another study found in the journal *Lancet,* researchers suggested that increased hydration actually increases the number of enzymes that cause fat burning. Last, a study found in the *European Journal of Clinical Nutrition* reaffirmed the effects of water on fat burning. The researchers found when the body is hydrated, fat is burned and muscle is preserved. Drinking water is definitely a must for sustainable fat loss and a healthy body composition.

5. Get eight hours of sleep. You feel terrible when you haven't gotten a good night's sleep, right? Well, there are a lot of benefits to be gained from a good night's sleep. When you fall asleep, your body releases growth hormone to help rebuild; it also helps to burn fat. Sleeping improves the immune system's ability to fight infection. It also reduces stress by lowering blood pressure and levels of stress hormones, elevated by our fast-paced lives. Sleep has also

been shown to regulate blood sugar, which can reduce your chance of developing diabetes.

Sleep regulates the appetite hormones leptin and ghrelin. Leptin signals the brain when your body has had enough food. Ghrelin stimulates hunger. A lack of sleep decreases leptin and increases ghrelin, which sets you up for an eating disaster. For most, this means eating high-calorie, low-nutrient-dense junk, which will make you fat. Besides putting your body composition at risk, sleep loss puts your health at risk. Facts found in *Brain, Behavior, and Immunity* and the *Archives of Internal Medicine*, state that sleep disturbance turns on genes that cause inflammation. During the inflammatory response, white blood cells produce inflammatory messengers called cytokines. Some cytokines communicate with other white blood cells to join in the inflammation; others, including IL-6, tumor necrosis factor, and C-reactive protein, are associated with a greater risk of developing heart disease, diabetes, certain cancers, obesity, and other inflammatory diseases, such as rheumatoid arthritis and Crohn's disease. Sleep loss was shown to increase IL-6, tumor necrosis factor and C-reactive protein. So, to keep your body fat down, and reduce your risk for developing chronic disease, get a good night's sleep—seven to eight hours is the target.

6. For some, eating legumes (beans) creates bloating and gas, making this nutritious food source a noisy nuisance. Legumes are an excellent source of carbs and protein, but unfortunately some people lack the enzyme alpha-galactosidase, which is needed to break down beans and cruciferous vegetables (broccoli, cauliflower, Brussels sprouts, and cabbage). After eating these food sources, bacteria in the gut help to break them down and produce large amounts of carbon dioxide and hydrogen. This causes the bloating, gas, and pain. The solution to this discomfort is to take a supplement containing the missing enzyme. The supplement I personally use is Carbo-G from Transformation Enzymes. It contains alpha-galactosidase, as well as other enzymes to help break down the annoying

proteins found in grains and beans. These digestive enzymes will help you break down beans and cruciferous vegetables, thus preventing the unpleasant symptoms.

7. Be careful with peanuts. As long as I'm discussing beans, I should warn you that a peanut allergy is a big deal. Peanuts actually are legumes (beans), not nuts. The problem for people who are allergic to peanuts is that they contain an insect-protective protein called lectin. Unlike other proteins, which are broken down during digestion, lectins aren't digested at all. They can attach to the intestine where immune cells are parked, waiting to attack invaders and unwanted proteins in our food. For many people, eating peanuts triggers the immune system to attack the lectins, causing an internal war, which can lead to conditions like leaky-gut syndrome, autoimmune conditions, and allergies. Second, peanuts can be contaminated during storage. Either from the soil or a poor storage environment, peanuts can be infected with a mold called Aspergillus Flavus. Aspergillus releases aflatoxin, a toxin which is not only carcinogenic (cancer causing), it also causes the nasty allergies associated with peanuts. Is it OK to eat them raw (i.e., raw peanut butter) or roasted? Either way—via mold or unwanted proteins—you're exposed to allergens (substances that cause the allergic response).

Why is the peanut-allergy epidemic so big now? Perhaps we introduce peanuts as a food source too early in life. Infants and children have an immature digestive system. Foreign proteins and other undesirable digested substances can get through the intestinal lining into the blood, where they have to face the immune system. The allergic response is then created by eating a food source not meant to be eaten at an early age; it should be postponed until the digestive system is able to handle these type of proteins. Also, there seems to be a growing consumption of peanuts; with more consumption there is a higher incidence of allergic reactions. My recommendation would be to abstain from feeding your children peanuts until they are three or four years old. If the digestive system can develop

Spice Up Your Diet!

FOOD	HERBS & SPICES
Poultry	Anise, black pepper, cayenne pepper, cardamom, celery seed, coriander, curry, fennel, garlic, ginger, lemon, marjoram, mustard, onion powder, oregano, paprika, red-pepper flakes, savory, sage, salt, thyme
Beef	Black pepper, cayenne pepper, chili powder, chipotle, curry, fenugreek, garlic, horseradish, mustard, onion, oregano, sage, salt, savory
Fish/Shellfish	Bay leaf, capers, dill, garlic, horseradish, lemon, marjoram, mustard, onion, parsley, rosemary, saffron, salt, tarragon, thyme
Stews & Soups	Bay leaf, Bragg Liquid Aminos, celery seed, chervil, chili powder, cilantro, cumin, curry, garlic, ginger, horseradish, marjoram, mustard, nutmeg, onion, oregano, paprika, parsley, saffron, salt, soy sauce (organic), thyme
Eggs	Basil, chervil, curry powder, dill, onion, paprika, pepper, rosemary, salt, tarragon, thyme
Vegetables	Basil, black pepper, cardamom, celery seed, chives, coriander, cumin, fennel, garlic, ginger, lemon, mint, onion, oregano, parsley, salt, sesame seed, thyme
Oatmeal	Allspice, anise, cinnamon, clove, cocoa (unsweetened), coconut, nutmeg, salt, vanilla

enough to take on these not-so-friendly food sources, we would probably see a tremendous drop in the number of people suffering from peanut allergies.

If you have a peanut allergy, you should stay away from them. Even if you aren't allergic to them, eat them sparingly. Better to eat nuts and seeds, including walnuts, macadamia nuts, pecans, pine nuts, pistachios, cashews, almonds, Brazil nuts, and pumpkin seeds.

OK, now take a breath. We just covered some great information about food. When you are putting in the effort to change your body composition, it's much easier when you know what's healthful and what's not. Too many times you and many others give up on "dieting" because it all gets confusing—and it can. Knowing what is good to eat is just as important as knowing what not to eat.

When you eat foods that are high in calories and low in nutrients, you turn on hormones that make you fat. In this next chapter, I'll show you which hormones create fat, and which ones burn fat. That's right. Those switches are fully under your control. I'm also going to show you a way to create a personalized, customized diet and food plan based on the needs of your body. Not only will you prevent and reverse chronic health problems; you will enjoy a leaner low-fat you.

D

I

ENJOY

T

Use the Right Switches

We have all heard the usual comments about dieting. It's going to be tough, boring, time-consuming, and, of course, the ever defeating "Forget it! It's just too damn hard to be healthy." Well, not this time. Yes, you have to change your inner dialogue and old, damaging habits. You need to be challenged to see yourself as worthy of being a healthier you. Unlike all the other diets and fads you may have followed, this time you don't have to give up amazing food, fun, and time in order to become lean and healthy from the inside out. This time you will use simple tools to empower yourself, have fun, feel energized, and, best of all, give yourself the gift of true, lasting health and vitality.

With the Body Composition Diet, you create a food plan that suits your specific physical needs, as well as an exercise program that fits your schedule. The key to a customized plan starts with an understanding of how your food choices affect your metabolism, your hormones, and your health. The foods you eat turn on certain hormones that regulate metabolism, store fat, and burn fat. These same foods also contain nutrients that regulate gene function to prevent and reverse chronic illness. Once you know this information, you can control your body composition. Like flipping on a light switch, you turn on the hormones responsible for making fat or burning it, as well as the genes that prevent and reverse disease.

Once you see how your hormones work, we are going to add in a few factors you need to know about yourself before you create your own diet. These factors include: body mass index, basal and total metabolic rates, and your body-fat percentage. These may sound complicated, but I have included simple equations to calculate each factor. You'll be

I Lost 45 Pounds, and My Blood Pressure is Normal

In August 2011, I visited my internist for my annual checkup. He told me to start blood-pressure and diabetes medications. I was angry because I had become diabetic, and because the internist offered no solutions other than pharmaceuticals. At the time, I was 53 years old, weighed 250 pounds, and thought I was eating the right foods to be healthy.

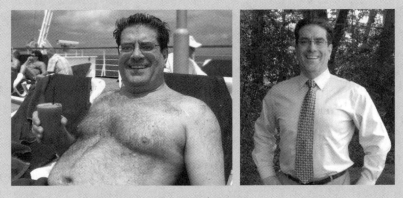

Before / After

At my first visit, Dr. Z ordered blood tests, conducted a body-fat analysis, and told me what foods to eat and what foods to avoid. He recommended nutritional supplements and taught me how to exercise properly using interval exercises for only 20 minutes a day. I have lost 45 pounds, significantly reduced my body fat, and my cholesterol levels and blood pressure are in the normal ranges. Also, I no longer suffer from sleep apnea. I feel like I'm 20 years old again. I feel like a poster boy for Dr. Z. I am always asked, "Tom, how did you lose all that weight? You look great!" My answer is simple: "It's a lifestyle change."

Dr. Z, thanks for saving my life!

Sincerely,

Tom M.

able to determine exactly how much food you need to eat daily in order to change your body composition.

In this chapter, I will provide sample diets to show you what a 1,300- and 1,500-calorie food plan looks like. By using the recipes at the end of the book, you can plug the calorie count right into your daily food plan. Or, you can choose foods you like from the lists I have provided to create your own meals and snacks.

You may have seen these equations elsewhere for calculating your BMI and body-fat percentage. What is new about this plan, compared to other diet programs, is that you will work smarter, not harder. You will choose the diet that fits your needs. Whatever diet you pick, you will not starve. You will not give up in frustration. You are going to see how these changes will affect your palate—and your health—for the better, and for the long run.

I know you are eager to get going. In the previous chapter I gave you the first of the three "Z Rules" to healthy and easy weight (fat) loss. Z Rule #1 was: Eat nutrient-dense, low-calorie foods. Here comes the second Z Rule.

Z Rule #2. Eat little to no carbs or large protein meals after 6–7 p.m.

I can hear the complaints now. "Huh? I can't do that. That's impossible. I don't get home until seven. What am I supposed to eat?" or "That's when my family eats dinner" or "I work late, so I eat late." OK, I know it sounds rough, but it's probably the single most powerful factor in losing fat—ever. The key to fat loss is not only to burn it or get rid of it, but also to stop making it. Our society is so crazed with losing weight that we will do anything to rid ourselves of it at any cost. We'll spend money on fad diets, fad weight-loss programs, the latest fat-sucking surgery, magic pills, creams, and elixirs. We'll starve ourselves to death and exercise ourselves into sheer exhaustion. Yet, if you want to lose the fat and restore your health, you must understand that food is like a control switch. Food not only provides us with energy; it also helps to regulate and control our hormones.

To master your body composition, you need to understand how to control these hormones. That's because certain hormones store fat, and others burn fat. Your fat-storing hormones include insulin, estrogen, and cortisol. Your fat-burning hormones include glucagon, HGH, testosterone, T3 (the most active thyroid hormone), and epinephrine. You may have heard of some of these, but even if you haven't, don't worry. The key hormones involved with storing or burning fat are only three: insulin, cortisol, and glucagon. I will also discuss the relationship between estrogen and body fat.

In our fast-paced society, the concept of eating small amounts of nutrient-dense foods throughout the day has been abandoned. Although humans are programmed to eat three meals a day, most people skip breakfast and eat their biggest meal at dinner. Most of us consume too much food, often containing the wrong types of calories. We aren't lions who kill and eat, then sleep for 10 to 12 hours. Evolutionally speaking, we are meant to graze—eat small meals often. Therefore, don't skip breakfast! According to research published in the *American Journal of Clinical Nutrition*, omitting breakfast impairs blood fats (triglycerides, HDL, and LDL) and causes you to gain weight (fat). Skipping breakfast because of "dieting"—or being too busy to eat—will send signals to your body that make you fat. Eat when you get up in the morning. Quick tip here: eat a breakfast that consists of protein, not high carbs. Research states that eating a protein breakfast not only controls your appetite; it turns off the hunger hormone ghrelin, and turns on the fat-burning hormone glucagon.

Here's the deal. While our bodies require a certain amount of food and calories to function properly, timing is everything. If you require 1,500 calories to sustain you through the day, what happens if you eat most of those calories at night? Those unused calories are stored as fat. While insulin is storing the fat, you also shut off the hormone that burns it—glucagon.

The release of these hormones is based on the type of foods you eat, the exercise you get, and the stress you endure. I want to emphasize the two major hormones that regulate, store, and burn fat—insulin and glucagon—so let's look at what they do inside the body.

Rich V. works in construction, mainly in stone and masonry. He's up at the crack of dawn and works till dusk. During his daily operations, he has to manage the job and oversee his crew, making sure they are doing a good job. He came to me because he was having a hard time managing his weight. With his long work hours, and the drive from job to job daily, he found it difficult to eat healthful foods at the most favorable times of the day. He sometimes skipped breakfast, ate bags of nuts—not a handful, but a bag—during the day, ate high-calorie foods for lunch, and then consumed far too much food at night before going to bed. Eating large amounts of protein and carbs late at night caused a surge of insulin that was released during his sleep. This resulted in a lot of excessive body fat.

After I gave him a plan, he was excited to make some changes. He began eating a healthful breakfast consisting of eggs mixed with vegetables, with sweet potato and fruit on the side. He took food to work to eat throughout the day. The biggest change was at night; he ate fewer carbs and less protein following his long day. In a few weeks, the belly fat came off. He had more energy to meet the demands of his job, as well as enough energy to get back to the gym.

Insulin is released into the blood mainly as a result of eating carbohydrates alone, or carbs combined with protein. When you eat carbs, your blood sugar goes up; this signals the pancreas to make insulin. Insulin takes sugar out of the blood and stores it in the liver and muscles as a substance called glycogen, which is a source of energy for the body. Once the liver and muscles are filled with glycogen, the rest of the blood sugar is stored as fat. Therefore, a rise in blood sugar produces a rise in insulin, which creates the potential for storing fat. Insulin is the fat-storage hormone.

Some functions of insulin are:

+ Insulin lowers blood sugar.

* Insulin shuttles sugar to the liver, muscles, and fat for energy.
* Insulin converts sugar and protein into fat.

Glucagon has the opposite effect. Glucagon is released when your blood sugar is low, as well as after eating protein. Eating protein stimulates the release of glucagon, which causes fat cells to release fat to be used for energy. By eating adequate amounts of protein, you can control glucagon levels during the day and night to help you get rid of fat. Even better, when you are not digesting food—i.e., when you are sleeping—you shut off insulin and release glucagon, allowing you to burn fat while you sleep. This causes the fat stores around your belly to be used for fuel. Glucagon is the fat-burning hormone.

Some functions of glucagon are:
* Glucagon raises blood sugar when it's low.
* Glucagon stimulates the release of fat to be burned for energy.
* Exercise stimulates the release of glucagon to burn fat.

Frank O. was fed up with his high cholesterol and LDL levels. He was frustrated with his weight and low energy. After I reviewed his blood work and lifestyle, it was clear that his current diet was making him sick and over-fat. We had to make some changes. First, he removed the refined carbs—white breads, pastas, and white rice—which produced higher-than-normal blood sugar and insulin. With too many of the wrong calories, insulin was storing his high blood sugar as fat. Second, we added three to four servings a day of protein from lean meat and fish. With each meal, he replaced simple carbs with sweet potato, wild rice, legumes, carrots, and beets. He also included dark leafy greens and vegetables with each meal. By eliminating the simple carbs and increasing his lean proteins, he reduced his blood sugar and insulin levels and increased his glucagon levels. To further stimulate the production of glucagon, Frank started high-intensity exercises three to four times a week. After implementing these simple steps, he proudly told me, "I have lost 30 pounds, cut my body-fat percentage in half, and lowered my cholesterol and blood pressure. I have more energy to do the things I enjoy outside of work."

FOOD COMBINATIONS AND THEIR EFFECT
ON INSULIN AND GLUCAGON LEVELS

Type of Food or Combination of Foods	Effect on Insulin	Effect on Glucagon	Effect on Fat Burning
Carbohydrate	++++	No change	Very Bad
Protein	++	++	Good
Fat	No change	No change	Good
Carb/Fat	++++	No change	Very Bad
Protein/Fat	++	++	Good
High Protein/Low Carb	++	++	Good
High Carb/Low Protein	++++++	+	Worst!

Individual foods, and foods in combination, affect insulin and glucagon levels. Remember, insulin stores fat, while glucagon burns fat. If you require 1,500 calories a day and you eat those calories during the day and not at night, you will turn on the fat-burning switch (glucagon) and burn fat while you sleep. If you eat lots of calories at night, insulin will cause those unused calories to be stored as fat while you sleep. Which do you want happening?

Have you ever heard of the sumo-wrestler diet? This is no joke. In order for sumo wrestlers to get as big and fat as they can, they consume roughly 20,000 calories a day. These calories are split into two meals followed by sleep. They skip breakfast and drink lots of beer (for added calories) with the monster meals. The sleep period causes the body to store this enormous caloric load as fat . . . lots of fat. Sadly, these wrestlers have a short life expectancy of 60 to 65 years due to their unhealthful lifestyle and the diseases (heart disease, high blood pressure, and diabetes) that develop from it.

The standard American diet is not too different, although I don't know anyone who eats 10,000-calorie meals. However, many people skip breakfast and then eat a couple of big meals later—the biggest one at dinner, fairly close to bedtime. Dinner is usually a combination of high-carb, low-protein foods. That combination sets you up for major fat storage at night, while you sleep—like a sumo wrestler, even though that's not what you're trying to do.

To lose weight (fat), you need to eat most of your food while the sun is out, and little to no food while the moon is out. If you eat dinner in the evening, choose foods that don't raise insulin: greens and non-starchy vegetables. Check the list at the end of this chapter. Dinner should consist of plenty of low-calorie greens with perhaps a tiny piece of protein (three ounces), along with a drop of olive oil and vinegar. Try a non-dairy vegetable soup, a tiny piece of flounder or tilapia, and a mixed-greens salad. You will find an endless number of foods you can use to create a low-calorie, non-insulin-raising meal. Later in this chapter, you will learn how to create a food plan specific to you, based on your caloric needs.

Before we turn away from insulin, I want to include a word to the wise for diabetics.

When trying to manage insulin resistance and diabetes, always combine a small amount of complex carbohydrates with a protein. This will produce a slow rise in blood sugar and, thus, a slow rise in insulin. The key to reversing blood-sugar spikes is to stop eating simple carbohydrates that flood your body with blood sugar. Eating mainly greens with lean protein and a small amount of slow-burning carbs, like sweet potato, squash, and beets, is the best way to regulate blood sugar.

Cortisol is the stress hormone. In times of stress, the brain tells the adrenal glands (located above the kidneys) to secrete cortisol. This hormone blocks inflammation and helps to regulate the allergic reaction. So what does this have to do with weight loss? When we restrict calories too much, blood-sugar levels drop. Cortisol is released into the body to help manage this blood-sugar loss. When blood sugars get too low, cortisol breaks down muscle to create sugar for the brain and nervous system. When you turn on this hormone, you are producing exactly the opposite of what you want for weight loss.

In stressful moments, cortisol helps the body deal with the stressors; this is a normal response. However, when stress is chronic, the prolonged release of cortisol can cause sleep issues, anxiety, muscle wasting, immune suppression, and an increase in belly fat. According to *Obesity Reviews*, chronic stress "inhibits the secretion of growth hormone, testosterone, and 17 beta-estradiol (estrogen), all of which counteract cortisol's effects. The net result is an accumulation of visceral fat." So, high cortisol from stress makes your belly fat. In another research article, from the journal *Psychosomatic Medicine*, researchers found that high cortisol levels cause circulating fat to be deposited deep in the abdomen. This is visceral fat, the dangerous fat. Visceral fat is linked to diabetes, heart disease, and cancers. In the next few pages, I've included a list of ways to help reduce stress and minimize the effects stress has on the body.

What is Stress?

You are sitting in an audience, and the speakers blast a high-pitched squeal—you cringe. You take your eye off the traffic light for a second, and the impatient driver behind you blasts the horn—your anger stirs. A police officer turns on the roof lights—your stomach twists. Last, an hour before that important exam, your stomach churns, rumbles, and you head for the bathroom due to GI distress. Sound familiar? We've all had a physical reaction to some experience. The experience is the stressor; the physical reaction is the stress reaction.

Stress is a perception or a momentary threat, which creates an adaptive response in the body to ensure survival—for example, shivering when you get cold, or sweating when you get too hot. The stressor can be physical (an infection, toxin or trauma) or emotional (abuse, guilt, fear, loss of a loved one, or any other source from work, home, or family). The stress reaction is the body's way of preparing itself for "fight or flight." Stress becomes a health hazard only when stressors are constant and the physical stress response doesn't stop. When we don't return to the normal pre-stress set point, the normal physical and emotional state, the result is disease.

Stress has always been considered a negative thing; in reality, it helps to maintain the natural workings of the body. There are positive stimuli that are considered stressors; exercise is the best example. This form of stimulus causes changes in the body to adapt to the demands of the physical activity. This form of stress has beneficial effects. The heart rate goes up; hormones are released to maintain blood sugar; and blood vessels dilate to send blood to the skeletal muscles to supply them with oxygen and glucose. There are many other reactions happening here, but you get my point. This type of stress is normal and natural. Once the physical activity stops, the body returns to a normal state of functioning.

Negative stimuli, like emotional stressors, also create changes in physiology in response to a specific event. Under emotional stress, the brain and body release hormones such as adrenaline, noradrenaline, and cortisol, along with other brain chemicals, as a response to the perceived threat or stressor. These acute stress reactions are momentary, or should be. Once the threat has passed, the body should come back to the normal state.

However, when the stress reaction becomes constant, disease can result. As stated previously, cortisol can suppress your immune system and decrease your ability to fight bacteria, viruses and cancer. The immune system is your internal armed services. When an invader, like a virus, enters the body, the body responds by sending out a type of white blood cell called a Natural Killer (NK) cell. Its role is to seek and destroy cancer cells, as well as those infected by viruses. Under prolonged stress, cortisol suppresses the function of the NK cell, thus allowing viruses to take hold and cancer cells to survive in the body. Individuals under constant stress often have outbreaks of shingles and/or cold sores; for some, stress causes the diagnosis or return of cancer. Cortisol is life-saving, but it can be a serious health hazard if not controlled.

In my case, there is no question that the stress I had, as well as my body's reaction, was a spark for the development of lymphoma. Emotional stress causes people to act in unfavorable ways. Under stress, we tend to eat processed, high-calorie foods in an attempt to make ourselves feel better. For me, the flood of stress hormones combined with a not-so-healthful diet set the stage for the creation of my disease.

Dr. Z's Tips to Keep Stress Under Control

Everyone experiences stress at times. The best way of dealing with it is to manage the stress as it occurs. Luckily, there are things you can do to reduce stress and prevent the health issues associated with long-term stress.

Relax. Relaxation is the opposite of stress, and it can create a sense of feeling calm. This can be accomplished simply by sitting quietly, doing slow, relaxed breathing, or participating in a few sessions of relaxing yoga.

Get a good night's sleep. Eight hours of good sleep each night increases healthy hormones like growth hormone (GH). GH helps to repair the body and regulates other hormones, which then control appetite. This is important because, without proper sleep, we tend to eat empty-calorie foods (simple carbohydrates) with no nutritional value. When we are under stress from life, the fight-and-flight reaction can cause damage to the body. A good night's sleep helps the body to repair after a stressful and busy day.

Eat healthful food. Stress causes malabsorption of nutrients from food, making nutrient-rich foods even more important. Food has a limitless supply of macro- and micro-nutrients to power us throughout the day, but most of us barely tap into this resource. We all can become more efficient eaters in order to function at our best. When we're stressed, it's easy to eat on the run or eat junk food or fast food. Yet, under stressful conditions, the body needs vitamins and minerals more than ever. For the sake of variety and health, a moderate diet consisting of protein, complex carbs, and good fats appears to be better in the long run. Frequent small meals allow a constant source of fuel for the body, which provides energy to power you through your day.

Get regular exercise. Research shows that regular exercise reduces the stress hormones adrenaline, norepinephrine, and cortisol. Exercise also boosts the immune system, increases healthy hormones, lowers blood pressure and cholesterol, and decreases the risk for developing cardiac disease, diabetes, and obesity. Different types of aerobic exercise can be performed for varying lengths of time, depending on how strenuous the activity is. Aerobic exercises include: dancing, skating, skiing, running, walking, bicycling, stair climbing, and swimming—high-intensity interval training.

Eliminate negativity. Create thoughts that build you up and give you abundance. Focus on situations you can control, and get rid of the negative people and talk in your life. Epigenetic research shows that we are our thoughts; what we focus on affects the physical body and internal environment. So think positively, and create your destiny.

Meditate. Meditation is a powerful tool for self-transformation. Scientists have found evidence that meditation has a biological effect on the body, changing the state of the brain and the autonomic (involuntary) nervous system. Researchers believe 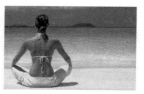 that these changes account for meditation's positive effects. The National Institutes of Health reports that regular meditation can reduce chronic pain, anxiety, blood pressure, substance abuse, post-traumatic stress response, and the blood levels of hormones.

Learning to manage stress is a lot more important than finding a way to mask it. Covering up stress with a crutch (i.e., alcohol, junk foods, medications, and destructive behaviors) to alleviate the outward symptoms will do little to help the situation get better. However, these simple methods for managing stress will help to eliminate it from your life.

Susan K. is an extremely active mother of two who works long hours and enjoys running and cycling. Prior to a scheduled orthopedic surgery, she came to see me with pain in her right shoulder and lower-right back. She also expressed frustration with fatigue, poor sleep, and difficulty dropping some unwanted body fat. Following her consultation, I ordered hormone testing and performed a physical and neurological exam on her to determine the cause of her pain. The hormone testing revealed high cortisol levels throughout the day and into the night. This explained her fatigue, poor sleep, and difficulty losing the fat. Although her diet was pretty good, we redesigned it to fit her lifestyle better. To control the cortisol and get her body to release glucagon, we increased her protein intake to three or four times a day. She replaced less desirable carbs with high-fiber carbs that didn't spike her blood sugar. Next, she ate before exercising and right after to replenish her energy—keeping her cortisol under control. Finally, she decreased the time she spent exercising and increased the intensity for shorter periods.

As a result, Susan was able to control her cortisol and increase her glucagon levels. In eight weeks she dropped 17 pounds of body fat, had more energy, and started to get a good night's sleep. Her shoulder pain and low-back pain were caused by unresolved muscle imbalances that required joint manipulation and therapeutic exercises. In less than four weeks she was 90 percent symptom free, and she canceled the unneeded surgery.

Estrogen, the third fat-storing hormone, is the main female sex hormone; it gives women their secondary sex characteristics and development of the reproductive organs. During and after menopause, estrogen levels drop. This causes fat to be stored in and around the belly, thighs, and buttocks. However, the relationship between estrogen and body fat is a double-edged sword.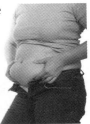
If estrogen levels plummet after menopause, you may store fat around the lower body. When there is excess body fat—for both women and men—estrogen levels can rise. Here's why. Fat tissue contains an enzyme called aromatase, which converts other hormones like testosterone into estrogen. When your body fat increases, so does aromatase activity and thus your levels of circulating estrogen. The consequences of high estrogen include uterine overgrowth (fibroids), breast cancer, infertility, impotence, prostatic enlargement, prostate cancer, thyroid dysfunction, high blood pressure, and more body fat. The good news is that eating a variety of whole foods and doing high-intensity exercise help to combat the effects of fat storage, and thus, maintain normal aromatase and estrogen levels.

To recap, the hormones that will make you fat are insulin, cortisol, and estrogen. The main hormone that will burn fat is glucagon. The better you know how your body works, the less frustration you will have with dieting to create the body you want.

The research is clear: the foods we eat and the types of exercise we get regulate the hormones that make us fat—and sick—as well as those that make us lean. In the "Transform" chapter, I will explain the most effective methods of exercising for maximum fat burning.

How Do You Measure Up?

Now that you know how to turn on and off the right switches in your body, you'll have a better understanding of the next section. You will see how you can calculate the diet plan that's just right for your body. By using a few powerful tools you will learn what you need to know about your body composition.

In my office I use a device called a bioelectrical body composition analyzer to measure body fat and lean muscle. The good news is that you don't need a machine to measure yourself. With a few simple calculations, you can determine your body-mass index—the relation of your weight to your height. From that you can determine your basal metabolic rate, which indicates how fast you can burn off weight when you are expending no energy at all. Finally, you'll come up with your body-fat percentage. These measurements will allow you to determine which diet is best for you. They also will give you a starting point, which then allows you to track your weight-loss progress along the way.

Body-Mass Index

BMI (body-mass index) is a tool that shows if you are a healthy weight for your height. It is also a way to calculate the health risk associated with your body composition—the ratio of lean tissues to fat. Determining your BMI is a simple calculation.

To calculate your BMI, divide your weight by your height squared. The units must be metric, so I'll also include how you can convert inches and pounds into their metric equivalents. The basic formula is:

BMI = Weight (kg) $\div$ Height in meters (m)^2

Let's use an example to see how this works. Say we have a person who weighs 160 pounds and is 5'8" (68") in height.

First we will convert the pounds to kilograms: Divide weight in pounds by 2.2.

160 lbs ÷ 2.2 = 73 kg (72.72 rounded off)

Now let's convert the inches to meters: Multiply height in inches by 2.54; then divide the total by 100. Multiply the resulting number by itself.

68" x 2.54 = 173 (172.72 rounded off)
173 ÷ 100 = 1.73 meters
1.73 x 1.73 = 2.99

Now let's combine those two numbers.

BMI = 73 ÷ 2.99 = 24.414

This person has a body-mass index of 24. A BMI of 20–25 is considered a normal weight. A BMI of 25–30 is considered overweight, and anything above 30 is obese. How did you measure up?

Body Mass Index Classifications		
Classification	**Risk**	**BMI Score**
Underweight	Moderate	Less than 18.5
Normal	Very low	18.5–24.9
Overweight	Low	25.0–29.9
Obese class 1	Moderate	30.0–34.9
Obese class 2	High	35.0–39.9
Extreme obesity	Very high	More than 40.0

Note: Someone who is overweight may not necessarily be "over-fat." A 5'5", 250-pound couch potato and a 5'5", 250-pound body builder have the same BMI. Why? BMI is merely the ratio of weight to height. It doesn't reveal if your weight is due to fat or muscle. That's what we're going to find out next.

Chart Your Progress

There's nothing better than before-and-after pix. Think of how proud you are when you renovate a room—or the whole house—and compare the wonderful changes to what was there before. Taking photos of yourself before you change will definitely be your best motivation not to go back. I suggest you take 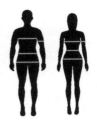 the photos three ways: from the front, from the side, and from the back. The pictures will be the proof of all your hard work.

Along with your BMI and body-fat percentage, physical measurements of your body will provide additional points of change and progress to keep you motivated. The best way to measure is without clothes. If you need someone to help you, you can wear a tank top and thin shorts, or something like that, to cover up. If you measure with clothes, remember to wear the *same* clothes each time you measure, so your values will be consistent.

Chest: Measure around your chest, across the nipple.

Waist: Measure around your waist, across your belly button (navel).

Hips: Measure around your hips and buttocks at the widest part.

Biceps: Measure the upper arm around the widest part of your bicep, *unflexed.*

After you take the "before" pictures, record your original BMI, body-fat percentage, and your measurements. At 4 weeks, 8 weeks and 12 weeks, record the measurements again to see how your body composition is improving. Continue recording your progress until you are satisfied with your results.

Start	4 Weeks	8 Weeks	12 Weeks
BMI	BMI	BMI	BMI
Body Fat	Body Fat	Body Fat	Body Fat
Chest	Chest	Chest	Chest
Waist	Waist	Waist	Waist
Hips	Hips	Hips	Hips
Biceps	Biceps	Biceps	Biceps
Weight	Weight	Weight	Weight

I have included weight as a measurement because it is important to use that as an additional marker of progress. Remember, the goal is to focus on losing the fat, while maintaining the lean muscle—not to focus solely on losing weight.

Basal Metabolic Rate

Now that you have your BMI, you need to calculate your basal metabolic rate (BMR). Your BMR is a calculation of your metabolism. You want your metabolism running high, because this will help you when you're dieting. Eating plenty of highly nutritious foods, along with exercise, speeds up metabolism. Starving yourself in the hope of fast fat loss slows down your metabolism. Why is that? Your body is developed from our ancient forebears, for whom a mastodon steak was not always available. Our bodies are genetically primed to store energy in case of starvation. When you starve yourself deliberately, you are telling your body to hold onto calories because food is not available. This causes fat burning to drop in order to conserve energy. And you are left wondering why you stopped losing fat.

Your Daily Energy Requirements

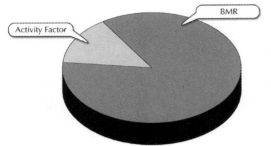

Basal Metabolic Rate
[calories your body burns for basic functions]

Activity Factor
[calories needed for movement and exercise]

The number of calories your body burns while at rest is called the basal metabolic rate. Everything you do takes effort—e.g., walking, reading, eating, and sleeping—and that burns calories. BMR is the amount of calories you would burn in a 24-hour period if your body were completely at rest. Once you figure out how many calories your body burns at a resting rate, you must then determine how active you are, which we will call the activity factor. On the next page, you can read about the activity factor, and how it affects your caloric needs. The BMR multiplied by the activity factor will result in a number we will call the total metabolic rate (TMR). Once the TMR is determined, you can calculate your percentage of body fat. Then you are ready to calculate how much food you need to eat in order to lose fat and put on muscle.

Basal Metabolic Rate Calculation
(from the Harris-Benedict Equation)

For women:

655 + (4.35 x weight in pounds) + (4.7 x height in inches) – (4.7 x age in years)

For men:

66 + (6.23 x weight in pounds) + (12.7 x height in inches) – (6.76 x age in years)

I'll use myself as an example. I'm 45 years old, 6' tall with a weight of 195 pounds. Before we start, let's convert that height into inches: 6 feet = 72 inches.

$$66 + (6.23 \times 195) + (12.7 \times 72) - (6.76 \times 45)$$
$$= 66 + 1214.85 + 914.4 - 304.2 = 1891.05$$

So my BMR would be 1891.05 while at rest. You try it: plug in your numbers and see what you get.

Activity Factor

In order for you to lose the fat, you have to know how many daily calories you need. Once you calculate your basal metabolic rate, you're ready to add an activity factor. Why is this necessary? Whether you are sedentary or very physically active, you are burning calories—just at different rates. The chart below gives some examples of what activities define each activity level. If you are active in some way, just compare it to what you see and figure out where you fall.

ACTIVITY ADJUSTMENT	
Sedentary or very light activity: Seated activities (computer work, reading, telephone work, driving), about 2 hours of walking/standing	Use BMR
Mild activity: Some walking throughout the day, standing activities (teaching, retail work), golf, light housework	1.2
Moderate activity: Fast walking, housework, gardening, carrying light loads, cycling, weight-lifting	1.3
Strenuous Activity: Dancing, skiing, physical labor (construction, moving cargo, road work), some running, very little sitting	1.5
Extreme activity: Endurance training, tennis, swimming, long-distance cycling/running, team sports (football, soccer, basketball)	1.7

Let's continue with myself as the example: I'm on my feet six to eight hours a day while in my practice, and I work out four to five days a week, performing 40 minutes of weights every other day and 20 minutes of high-intensity interval training on the other days. Due to my busy work week, sometimes I miss a day or two. I would classify my activity level at strenuous (1.5).

My BMR (1891.05) x my activity level (1.5) = 2,836 calories; this is my total metabolic rate (TMR). This is how many calories I require every day to maintain a healthy body composition. If I wanted to lose body fat, I would take certain steps. One of them would be to reduce the number of calories ever so slightly. This would help to regulate insulin and cause the fat to start coming off. The next step would be to exercise with intensity, which causes an increase in the fat-burning hormone glucagon. That increases lean muscle, which acts as a fat furnace and prevents the hormone insulin from storing more fat.

> Ryan was training for the armed services. He was thin and strong, but was unable to increase his weight no matter what he tried. After consulting with him, I had him fill out a seven-day food diary before sitting with him to calculate how much food he needed based on his physical demands. Through the use of bioelectrical impedance and from his current diet, we determined he was clearly not eating enough to match his activity level. Training for the armed services can be grueling. We rated his activity as a 1.7. That meant the amount of food he needed should be doubled. Because he had no fat to lose, there were no calories taken away from his diet. In three months, he reported putting on 12 pounds—mission accomplished.

Body-Fat Percentage Calculation

There are different methods for measuring body fat. The most accurate and cost-effective way is to be tested via bioelectrical impedance. However, to give you a general sense of your body-fat percentage, researchers have created another formula. It will not calculate the exact percentage, but it will give you a guideline as you go forward to determine if you are losing body fat and/or muscle. The equation below is called the Jackson-Pollock formula.

Adult Body Fat % = (1.61 x BMI) + (0.13 x Age) – (12.1 x your gender) – 13.9

Gender values: men = 1, women = 0

Jackson-Pollock Body-Fat Percentage Charts

If you have the ability to get your body fat tested via bioelectrical impedance, again, you will have a more accurate body-fat value. You can also buy body-fat calipers that use skin-fold testing. This method involves pinching the skin and fat over different parts of your body, putting roughly seven measurements into a formula to calculate your fat percentage. You can also use the formula I have provided. The Jackson-Pollock formula is just a formula, but at least it gives you a starting point to later revisit in order to chart your progress.

Once you have calculated your body-fat percentage, look at the charts provided to see where you fall. One chart is for men and the other for women. Your percentage will indicate whether you are at a healthy fat level. For a 45-year-old woman, a body-fat percentage between 23 percent and 28 percent is ideal, whereas between 29 percent and 34 percent is average.

As you can see on the charts, with age the body-fat percentage goes up. As we age, physical and metabolic changes take place that increase body fat. This increased fat is sometimes seen around the organs (visceral fat) and within the muscles (intramuscular fat). Once you have calculated your TMR and your body-fat percentage, you can determine how many calories to cut from your diet in order to start losing fat.

Insulin, cortisol, and glucagon are the hormones that dictate your body composition, whether you get fat or lean. These three hormones are also influenced by the foods you eat and the combinations of these foods. Carbs alone, and a combination of high carbs and low protein, seem to have the most influence on expanding your waistline. Understanding

BODY FAT % MEASUREMENT CHART FOR WOMEN

AGE																	
18-20	11.3	13.5	15.7	17.7	19.7	21.5	23.2	24.8	26.3	27.7	29.0	30.2	31.3	32.3	33.1	33.9	34.6
21-25	11.9	14.2	16.3	18.4	20.3	22.1	23.8	25.5	27.0	28.4	29.6	30.8	31.9	32.9	33.8	34.5	35.2
26-30	12.5	14.8	16.9	19.0	20.9	22.7	24.5	26.1	27.6	29.0	30.3	31.5	32.5	33.5	34.4	35.2	35.8
31-35	13.2	15.4	17.6	19.6	21.5	23.4	25.1	26.7	28.2	29.6	30.9	32.1	33.2	34.1	35.0	35.8	36.4
36-40	13.8	16.0	18.2	20.2	22.2	24.0	25.7	27.3	28.8	30.2	31.5	32.7	33.8	34.8	35.6	36.4	37.0
41-45	14.4	16.7	18.8	20.8	22.8	24.6	26.3	27.9	29.4	30.8	32.1	33.3	34.4	35.4	36.3	37.0	37.7
46-50	15.0	17.3	19.4	21.5	23.4	25.2	26.9	28.6	30.1	31.5	32.8	34.0	35.0	36.0	36.9	37.6	38.3
51-55	15.6	17.9	20.0	22.1	24.0	25.9	27.6	29.2	30.7	32.1	33.4	34.6	35.6	36.6	37.5	38.3	38.9
56 & up	16.3	18.5	20.7	22.7	24.6	26.5	28.2	29.8	31.3	32.7	34.0	35.2	36.3	37.1	38.1	38.9	39.5
	LEAN			IDEAL			AVERAGE					ABOVE AVERAGE					

BODY FAT % MEASUREMENT CHART FOR MEN

AGE																	
18-20	2.0	3.9	6.2	8.5	10.5	12.5	14.3	16.0	17.5	18.9	20.2	21.3	22.3	23.1	23.8	24.3	24.9
21-25	2.5	4.9	7.3	9.5	11.6	13.6	15.4	17.0	18.6	20.0	21.2	22.3	23.3	24.2	24.9	25.4	25.8
26-30	3.5	6.0	8.4	10.6	12.7	14.6	16.4	18.1	19.6	21.0	22.3	23.4	24.4	25.2	25.9	26.5	26.9
31-35	4.5	7.1	9.4	11.7	13.7	15.7	17.5	19.2	20.7	22.1	23.4	24.5	25.5	26.3	27.0	27.5	28.0
36-40	5.6	8.1	10.5	12.7	14.8	16.8	18.6	20.2	21.8	23.2	24.4	25.6	26.5	27.4	28.1	28.6	29.0
41-45	6.7	9.2	11.5	13.8	15.9	17.8	19.6	21.3	22.8	24.7	25.5	26.6	27.6	28.4	29.1	29.7	30.1
46-50	7.7	10.2	12.6	14.8	16.9	18.9	20.7	22.4	23.9	25.3	26.6	27.7	28.7	29.5	30.2	30.7	31.2
51-55	8.8	11.3	13.7	15.9	18.0	20.0	21.8	23.4	25.0	26.4	27.6	28.7	29.7	30.6	31.2	31.8	32.2
56 & up	9.9	12.4	14.7	17.0	19.1	21.0	22.8	24.5	26.0	27.4	28.7	29.8	30.8	31.6	32.3	32.9	33.3
	LEAN			IDEAL			AVERAGE					ABOVE AVERAGE					

how to measure your metabolism and how much food you need is just as important as knowing what hormones are turned on by what kinds of foods. The key to sustainable dieting is having control over your hormones, metabolism, and the food choices you make.

Now let's turn to the part you've been waiting for. Let me show you how to create a diet that is custom-made for you. You'll learn how many calories suit what you're trying to do for yourself. Then you'll see how many delicious ways you can prepare food that makes your body want to sing!

Your Custom-Made Diet

Here's a cool concept: a diet program personalized and customized—tailored to you. The old saying, "No two people are alike," is the truth. In conversation you frequently hear, "My grandfather ate crap and drank his whole life and never got sick," or "That person never smoked a cigarette in his life and developed lung cancer," and "Why does she get to eat whatever she wants and not gain a pound?" How can this be? Simply, each person, including you, has a unique genetic blueprint that defines who you are. What you look like, how fast you heal, how you respond to stress, and how well your body manages the calories you take in from food—all are unique to you. So, how can we all follow the same diet? A diet that works for one person may not work for you. The same goes for exercises. The ones that come out of a box or DVD jacket may burn fat for some and not others. I hope you get my point.

The key is to fill your plate with nutrient-dense foods without loading up on calories. How much do you eat? I have included an example of a meal plan for one day based on two different caloric requirements. You'll also notice that I suggest you eat five to six times a day, so the chart has three meals and three snacks. Following my example, there is a blank sheet for you to use to make up your target daily caloric intake.

Don't forget to fill your plate with colorful vegetables each time you eat; they're listed under Non-Starchy Vegetables. Those foods are loaded with fiber and water, both of which will satisfy your hunger and provide you with nutrients to aid digestion, regulate hormones, and, most important, reverse and rebuild from disease.

Your three meals should consist of dark-green and rainbow-colored vegetables and protein. Depending on your caloric

I Lost 17 Pounds and Fixed My Hormones

For 18 months I suffered from chronic shoulder issues; the diagnosis was a sprain/strain of the rotator cuff. After countless hours of physical therapy, I no longer hoped for a full recovery. As an athlete, I trained around my injury. I visited several reputable orthopedic doctors who recommended surgery for my shoulder and steroids for my hip and back.

At my first appointment, Dr. Zembroski (Dr. Z) conducted a full muscular, skeletal, and neurological evaluation. He immediately found the root cause of my issues. The entire right side of my body was weak, causing my shoulder and back problems. No other physician had taken the time to figure out what actually caused my problems.

With a full nutritional and body-composition evaluation, I was able to stabilize my hormones and alleviate symptoms of arthritis. Dr. Z provided nutritional supplements to decrease joint inflammation and lower my levels of cortisol—a hormone linked to cancer and other chronic diseases. Using food and lifestyle changes, I was able to lose 17 pounds in eight weeks, while significantly increasing my lean-muscle mass.

I can only describe my experience, and the level of care in his office, as life-changing.

—Susan K.

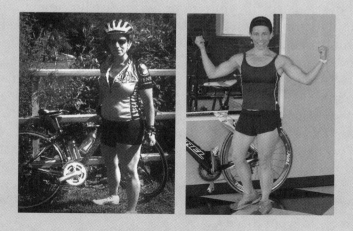

Before / After

needs, you may include a high-fiber starchy carbohydrate, and a fat. The snack sections should include the other food groups including nuts/seeds, legumes, limited choice of grains, and fruits. Don't forget the facts about peanuts and legumes from the previous chapter.

Step by Step

Now let's put it all together. Your total metabolic rate is the number of calories that serve as your baseline. From this number, you need to decide how many calories to subtract from your total metabolic rate to start getting rid of the fat. Use the chart below to determine how many calories to subtract. The key here is not to severely restrict calories. You want to take away a small amount of calories, so you don't release cortisol and hold onto the fat. Fat loss is a process, not an event.

FAT-LOSS ADJUSTMENT	
Men:	
If you have a healthy body-fat percentage:	No subtraction of calories
If you have an increased body-fat percentage:	Subtract 200–500 calories
If your body-fat percentage is more than 30%:	Subtract 300–600 calories
Women:	
If you have a healthy body-fat percentage:	No subtraction of calories
If you have an increased body-fat percentage:	Subtract 100–300 calories
If your body fat percentage is more than 35%:	Subtract 300–500 calories

Here's another way to think about it. One person's fat-loss needs are different than another's fat-loss needs. If person A had a body-fat percentage of more than 30 percent, subtracting 300 to 600 calories would be appropriate. If person B had a slight increased body-fat percentage, subtracting the same 300 to 600 calories would be too drastic. The point is to modify your caloric intake based on *your* metabolic rate and body-fat percentage. This makes dieting customized and tailored to you.

Now, calculate how much food in calories you need to eat daily. Multiply your basal metabolic rate by the activity adjustment. This becomes your total metabolic rate. Subtract the calories from the fat-loss adjustment table from your total metabolic rate. This is your daily caloric intake.

CALCULATE YOUR DAILY CALORIC INTAKE	
Basal Metabolic Rate (BMR):	
Activity Adjustment:	X
Total Metabolic Rate:	
Fat-Loss Adjustment:	−
Your Daily Caloric Intake*	=

*This is the amount of food you eat each day.

Let's use Sue's calculations as an example. Her BMR after calculations was 1,280. She cycles a few days a week, not for competition, but to enjoy the outdoors and the exercise, and works out with weights when she can another few days a week. Along with her exercising, she has an active career. I would give her an activity factor of 1.3. Her total metabolic rate is 1,664. This is the number of calories her body needs to sustain normal function and maintain her current body composition. However, her body-fat percentage at 41 years old was about 31 percent. Looking at the fat-loss adjustment chart, we decided to subtract 300 calories from her daily intake. Her daily caloric intake is 1,364 calories.

How to Choose Your Foods

Let's say that your daily caloric needs are about 1,300 calories. There are a couple of ways to do this. The first is to use the optimal-foods lists at the end of this chapter. When deciding what to eat, or how much, note how many calories each food provides. For example, two whole eggs are 150 calories, while one-half cup of sweet potato is 125 calories. You can create your own meals and snacks from the optimal foods that fit your specific caloric needs. Serving sizes and their respective calories are already calculated for you. You just decide what you like to eat. The second way is to use the recipes in the back of the book. There, too, the calories per serving have been calculated. If you like to make super-tasty meals loaded with nutrients, this may be your method. While some of these recipes take a few minutes to prepare, others take very little time. See Dr. Z's Fast Food on page 80 for ideas. Many of the foods on the optimal-foods lists and in the recipes at the back of the book are "grab and go" food items. Depending on your lifestyle, you pick the foods and recipes convenient for you. If you choose a recipe that requires preparation time, save time by making enough for leftovers. Perhaps you cook a lot on a Sunday, and eat the leftovers for the next couple of days.

Using the optimal-foods lists, fill in the worksheet with your choices. Each meal should have protein, some carbs, some fat, and lots of non-starchy vegetables. See the example written up for 1,300 calories.

If your total metabolic rate requires you to eat 1,300 calories, then it's 1,300 you eat. This is a custom food plan for you—like a custom-made suit or a ring that fits just right. It may seem like a lot of food, but don't forget, the foods you are now eating are high in nutrients and low in calories. So you are consuming more than you were in the past. Eat most of the food during the day and less at night. If you eat dinner late, I suggest a small piece of protein and hearty portion of greens. If you are hungry at night, eat vegetables with few calories and lots of nutrients. Remember, you don't want to store fat while sleeping, so don't eat foods that raise insulin. Stick to non-starchy vegetables, like Brussels sprouts, bell peppers, or cucumber, to satisfy your hunger.

The recipes in the back of the book will provide you with meals that you can plug right into your custom calorie requirements. The following shows the 1,300-calorie meal-planning worksheet filled with the meals from the recipes.

The additional snacks are whatever you decide. The calories in this example add up to roughly 1,361 calories. Don't drive yourself crazy when putting your meals together. Try to get as close to your calorie requirements as possible.

Now let's take a look at a meal plan that consists of 1,500 calories. Let's set it up the same way we did with the 1,300-calorie meal plan by using the optimal foods lists, and then using recipes from the back of the book. You can use your own recipes as well. Just be sure to go through the ingredients in your recipes to calculate the calories per ingredient, and then divide the total calories by the number of servings to get the calories per serving. Here is a website that is a good resource to help you calculate calories: www.nutritiondata. self.com. This approach requires a little bit of work at first, but it makes your dieting adventure easy and enjoyable.

NOTE: When using your own recipes, or recipes you find elsewhere, be sure to replace unhealthful ingredients with healthful ones so you are not eating too many calories or the wrong kind of calories. For example, if you are used to eating regular white or wheat pasta, replace it with brown-rice pasta. In salad dressings, use only cold-pressed olive oil, not regular vegetable oils. When frying eggs or sautéing onions, use grapeseed oil instead of vegetable oil. If a recipe calls for cow milk, substitute non-dairy milk from the optimal foods lists. At the end of this section, you will find a list of foods to avoid.

The 1,500-calorie pick-and-place meal plan worksheet shows that creating a day's worth of meals is fairly simple, customized, and . . . you get to eat a lot of food. There are no restrictions, except the foods to avoid—the ones that will make you fat and unhealthy. Using the recipes again, fill in the meals and snacks for a 1,500-calorie per day requirement.

MEAL PLANNING WORKSHEET

1,300 CALORIES	
MORNING MEAL Protein: **2 whole eggs** Carb: **1/2 sweet potato** Fat: **1 tsp grapeseed oil** Additional Foods: **1 serving non-starchy vegetables** **1 cup blueberries**	Start your day with protein: eggs, veggie burger, chicken. Add a complex carb, some fat, and a non-starchy vegetable. Include a fruit. Eat most of your food during the day, not at night.
SNACK **10 almonds** **1 medium apple** **1/2 cup carrots**	8–10 almonds is the limit. No need to overeat at snack time.
MIDDAY MEAL Protein: **3–4 oz chicken** Carb: **1/2 cup brown rice with black beans** Fat: **1/4 avocado** Additional Foods: **1 serving non-starchy vegetables**	Pick another protein: turkey burger, chicken salad, or chicken with green salad and 1/4 avocado (2 servings). Another non-starchy vegetable, and legumes on the side.
SNACK **6–8 brown-rice crackers** **1/4 cup hummus**	Remember: Eat most of your calories before dark.
EVENING MEAL Protein: **3–4 oz fish** Carb: **1/2 cup lentil soup** Fat: **1 tsp olive oil** Additional Foods: **1 serving non-starchy vegetables**	Low calories now. Small cup of bean soup; 3 ounces baked or broiled fish with spices, 1/2 cup of sweet potatoes; Brussels sprouts or steamed broccoli.
SNACK **Non-starchy vegetable** **Herbal tea**	If you're hungry, eat half a cucumber or red bell pepper.

MEAL PLANNING WORKSHEET

1,300 CALORIES	
MORNING MEAL **Scrambled Eggs with Sundried Tomatoes** **1/2 cup of Strawberries and 1/2 cup of Blueberries** **1/2 cup of Roasted Brussels Sprouts with Shallots**	Eggs with sundried tomatoes provide 318 calories. Berries have about 75 calories. Sundried tomatoes and oil to cook eggs provide some fat.
SNACK **1 medium apple** **6–8 ounces fresh-brewed unsweetened green tea**	An apple has 70 calories, and the tea has no calories. Green tea is a great fat burner!
MIDDAY MEAL **Ground Turkey Bolognese** **Mixed Green Salad with 1 teaspoon vinaigrette**	This meal includes protein, fat, and carb (brown-rice pasta) with about 392 calories. The oil in the salad has 40 calories.
SNACK **1 cup of Broccoli** **1/4 cup of Hummus**	Broccoli with hummus provides about 120 calories.
EVENING MEAL **Salmon Salad with sliced cucumbers and tomatoes** **Pantry Salad**	This meal includes protein, fat, and carbs. Salmon Salad has 186 calories. The Pantry Salad and dressing are 110 calories.
SNACK **Tomato with fresh basil and a few drops of olive oil** **Herbal tea**	This has about 50 calories.

MEAL PLANNING WORKSHEET

1,500 CALORIES	

MORNING MEAL
Protein: **3 egg whites &**
   1 whole egg
Carb: **1/2 sweet potato**
Fat: **2 tsp grapeseed oil**
Additional Foods: **1 serving**
   non-starchy vegetables
1 cup mixed berries
	Egg whites plus a whole egg provide 150 calories. Add chopped spinach or collard greens. Sweet potato and oil for frying provide 205 calories. Berries have 75 calories.

SNACK **10 almonds** **1 medium apple** **1/2 cup of carrots**	Almonds, apple, and 1/2 cup of carrots provide 225 calories.
MIDDAY MEAL Protein: **3–4 oz chicken** Carb: **1 medium carrot** Fat: **1 tbsp oil** Additional Foods: **1 serving** **non-starchy vegetables**	Grilled chicken over green salad with a medium shredded carrot and olive-oil dressing provide a total of 300 calories.
SNACK **1 brown-rice cake** **1 tbsp of almond butter**	This combination provides 135 calories.
EVENING MEAL Protein: **3–4 oz fish** Carb: **1/2 cup lentil soup** Fat: **1 tbsp olive oil** Additional Foods: **1 serving** **non-starchy vegetables**	3–4 ounces wild salmon baked or broiled with lemon and dill; 1/2 cup lentil soup; and green salad with olive-oil vinaigrette provide a total of 385 calories.
SNACK **Red and yellow bell peppers** **Herbal tea**	Depending on the amount you eat, this has 25–50 calories.

MEAL PLANNING WORKSHEET

1,500 CALORIES	
MORNING MEAL **Feisty Breakfast Medley** **Fresh-brewed green tea**	This provides protein, carb, and fat in one dish for 217 calories.
SNACK **Ambrosia Fruit Salad**	The fruit and coconut will satisfy your sweet tooth for 188 calories.
MIDDAY MEAL **Curried Chicken Salad** **Baked Sweet Potato Cubes**	Chicken salad provides 367 calories. The sweet potatoes add 123 calories.
SNACK **Broccoli and Hummus**	One cup provides 139 calories.
EVENING MEAL **Summer Poached Salmon** **Pantry Salad**	One serving provides 359 calories. Use the salad recipe, or what you have on hand. Calories should be about 110.
SNACK **Choose a non-starchy vegetable**	Tomatoes and cucumbers have about 50 calories.

The total calorie count of the recipes and meals is 1,553. Now, if you remember from the beginning, I said you wouldn't have to count calories; you don't. The calorie counting has already been done for you. You just pick what you want to eat, and plug in the individual foods or recipes. The important thing to remember is portion control. When eating protein, common sense tells us not to eat a 12–16-ounce steak, just as eating an entire pound of nuts is too extreme. The following pictures provide a visual reference to common portion sizes.

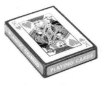 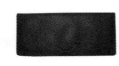

| 3-4 oz piece of meat or chicken (deck of cards) | 3-4 oz piece of fish (small checkbook) | 1 cup (baseball) | 1/2 cup (lightbulb) | 1 tablespoon (poker chip) |

If you can remember a few images, figuring out how much to eat of something becomes very simple: no points, no scales, no guesswork. You don't need to get out the calculator when trying to determine portion sizes. Here's another way to think about portion size. The right amount of protein for you is the size of your palm; a serving of carbs should be roughly the size of your clenched fist. The point here is to have an idea, so you don't overeat calories.

In the recipe section, you'll be pleasantly surprised to see there are fun things to prepare and enjoy. Flourless almond-butter cookies and gluten-free banana muffins are delicious! These are treats to enjoy as you hit your goals. Now let's talk about alcohol.

Alcohol—in the form of wine, beer, or spirits—has calories. The body breaks down alcohol into a vinegar-like substance called acetate, which, in turn, must be processed. This slows down the burning of fat, causing you to hold onto it. The second problem with alcohol is the "munchy" factor. I'm sure most of us have gotten the munchies after having a drink or two. Food has calories, and alcohol has calories. When do most people drink alcohol? At night. Drinking before, during, or after dinner turns on the fat-making process. If you are in the habit of drinking alcohol at night and you can't seem to get rid of belly bulge, you may want to reconsider that cocktail.

On page 148 is a blank meal-planning worksheet for you to work with. Remember to have a few servings each day of protein, carbs, and fat. Eat green leafy vegetables five to six times a day to get vitamins, minerals, fiber, and water.

"Foods" to Avoid

Dairy

Milk, yogurt, cheese, ice cream, etc. It doesn't matter if the milk is from cows, goats, or sheep. Dairy products are inflammatory, and most contain traces of hormones and antibiotics. Even organic milk products may contain somatic cells—white blood cells that fight infection in the cows' udders and get passed on to the consumer. Instead, use rice milk, almond milk, and coconut milk. Coconut-milk yogurt and ice cream are becoming widely available.

Sugar

Sugar goes by many different names. Read labels, and avoid foods containing the following: barley malt, blackstrap molasses, brown sugar, cane sugar, confectioner's sugar, corn sweetener, corn syrup, date sugar, dextrin, dextrose, d-mannose, evaporated cane juice, fruit-juice concentrate, glucose, high-fructose corn syrup (HFCS), honey, lactose, malt syrup, maltodextrin, maltose, maple syrup, molasses, raw sugar, sucrose, syrup, table sugar, turbinado sugar.
NOTE: *Fructose, naturally occurring in fruit or added in small quantities to foods, is acceptable.*

Grains

Most grains contain gluten, gliadin, or lectins and are major sources of inflammation. Even whole grains contain indigestible protein, which can be detrimental for those with gluten or gliadin sensitivities. The only grains acceptable are brown rice, quinoa, steel-cut oats, and wild rice.

Meat/Eggs/Fish

Beef, poultry, and eggs raised on factory farms which use grain feed, antibiotics, and hormones.
NOTE: *Look for grass-fed beef raised without antibiotics or hormones, free-range poultry, and organic, farm-fresh eggs.*

Farm-raised fish, which may contain petroleum dyes used for coloring.
NOTE: *Look for wild-caught seafood.*

Cured meats (deli, sausages, bacon), especially those containing nitrates.

NOTE: *Packaged turkey bacon or chicken/turkey sausage should be organic and natural with no preservatives or sugar.*

Fats/Oils

Margarine and other butter substitutes; partially hydrogenated vegetable oils; aerosol cooking sprays, such as PAM; and trans-fats (synthetic fats found in many processed foods).

NOTE: *Foods labeled "0 Trans Fats" may, by law, contain small amounts of trans fats. Look for foods labeled "No Trans Fats" or "Trans-Fat Free."*

Processed Foods

Processed peanut butter—most contain hydrogenated oil, sugar, and preservatives.

Canned foods, unless both unsweetened and organic.

NOTE: *Try to find products in cans labeled "BPA-free."*

Soda and energy drinks, including "diet" versions and any beverage containing more than 10 calories.

Artificial sweeteners, such as saccharine, sucralose, and aspartame.

Artificial flavors, food dyes, and coloring.

NOTE: *Try to eat whole-food sources and/or organic packaged foods with natural ingredients.*

MEAL PLANNING WORKSHEET

_____ CALORIES	
MORNING MEAL Protein: Carb: Fat: Additional Foods:	
SNACK	
MIDDAY MEAL Protein: Carb: Fat: Additional Foods:	
SNACK	
EVENING MEAL Protein: Carb: Fat: Additional Foods:	
SNACK	

OPTIMAL FOODS

PROTEIN	3 Servings Per Day

Animal Sources — Serving = 150 calories

Choose free-range, cage-free, grass-fed with no hormones or antibiotics added. Avoid farm-raised fish.
Poultry, lean (3–4 oz) Chicken • Turkey — **Cold-Water Fish** (3 oz or 3/4 cup canned in water) Cod • Halibut • Mackerel • Salmon • Tuna — **Shellfish** (3 oz or 3/4 cup canned in water) Crab • Lobster • Shrimp — **Red Meat**, lean (3–4 oz) Beef, steak or ground • Lamb — **Game** (3–4 oz) Buffalo • Ostrich • Venison — **Eggs** (2 whole or 3 whites + 1 whole)

Plant Sources — Calories per serving vary

Soy or "Veggie" burger, gluten-free (4 oz = 100) • Tempeh (1/2 cup = 165) • Tofu (1/2 cup fresh = 183)

NON-STARCHY	Unlimited Servings, minimum 3-4

Serving = approximately 10–25 calories   *Use raw, cooked, or juiced*

Arugula • Asparagus • Bamboo Shoot • Bean Sprout • Beet Green • Bell Pepper • Bok Choy • Broccoli • Broccoflower • Brussels Sprout • Cabbage (all types) • Cauliflower • Celery • Chicory • Chive • Collard Green • Cucumber • Dandelion Green • Eggplant • Endive • Escarole • Fennel • Garlic • Green Bean • Heart of Palm • Jalapeño Pepper • Kale • Leek • Lettuce (all types)• Mushroom (all types) • Mustard Green • Okra • Onion • Radicchio • Radish • Romaine • Scallion • Shallot • Snow Pea • Spinach • Swiss Chard • Spaghetti Squash • Summer Squash • Tomato • Water Chestnut • Watercress • Zucchini

HIGH-FIBER STARCHY	3 Servings Per Day

Serving = 1/2 cup

Acorn Squash (56) • Artichoke Heart (42) • Beet (37) • Butternut Squash (40) • Carrot (27, or 2 raw = 50, 1/2 cup baby = 30) • Pumpkin (142) • Sweet Potato (125) • Turnip (17) • Winter Squash (40) • Yam (79)

OPTIMAL FOODS

LEGUMES
Serving = 1/2 cup
Adzuki Bean (147) • Black Bean (114) • Chickpea (Garbanzo) (134) • Edamame (127) • Great Northern Bean (104) • Green Pea (62) • Hummus (208) • Kidney Bean (112) • Lentil (115) • Lima Bean (108) • Mung Bean (80) • Navy Bean (127) • Pinto Bean (122) • White Bean (110)

GRAINS
Serving = 45 calories
Brown Rice, all types (1/2 cup cooked = 108) • Brown-Rice Cracker (6 = 160) • Brown-Rice Cake (2 = 70) • Oatmeal, steel-cut (1/2 cup cooked = 150) • Pasta, brown-rice (2 oz cooked = 210) • Quinoa (1/2 cup cooked = 111) • Wild Rice (1/2 cup cooked = 83)

FATS / OILS	3 Servings Per Day
Serving size and calories vary	

Use grapeseed oil for cooking; it has a very high smoke point. Use olive oil for salads and adding flavor to cooked foods.

Almond, dry-roasted (2 Tbsp = 100) • Avocado (1/8 = 40) • Cashew, dry-roasted (2 Tbsp = 100) • Coconut, unsweetened (2 Tbsp = 100) • Coconut Milk (1-1/2 Tbsp = 40) • Coconut Milk Creamer, unsweetened (1 Tbsp = 10) • Hazelnut, raw (2 Tbsp = 90) • Macadamia Nut, dry-roasted (1 Tbsp = 60) • Mayonnaise (1 Tbsp = 48) • Nut Butter (1 Tbsp = 100) • Oils—canola, coconut, flaxseed, grapeseed, olive, peanut (1 tsp = 40) • Olive (8–10 medium = 40) • Pecan, dry-roasted (2 Tbsp = 100) • Peanut, dry-roasted (2 Tbsp = 100) • Pistachio, raw (2 Tbsp = 85) • Vegenaise® (1 Tbsp = 90) • Walnut, raw (2 Tbsp = 100)

OPTIMAL FOODS

DAIRY ALTERNATIVES

Serving size and calories vary

Almond Milk, unsweetened (1 cup = 50) • Coconut Milk Beverage, unsweetened (1 cup = 50) • Coconut Milk Yogurt, unsweetened (4 oz = 80) • Hemp Milk, unsweetened (1 cup = 130) • Rice Milk, unsweetened (1 cup = 70)

FRUITS

Serving size and calories vary

Choose whole fruit rather than juice. Juice has a much higher glycemic index because the fiber has been removed.

Low Glycemic Index: Berries (1 cup)—Blackberry (62) • Blueberry (84) • Boysenberry (166) • Cranberry (46) • Elderberry (106) • Gooseberry (66) • Loganberry (81) • Raspberry (64) • Strawberry (50)

Medium Glycemic Index: Apple (1 = 95) • Apricot (1 = 17) • Cherry (15 = 75) • Grapefruit (1 = 82) • Kiwi (1 = 50) • Lemon/Lime (1 = 17) • Melon (slice = 50) • Nectarine (1 = 62) • Orange (1 = 62) • Passion Fruit (1 = 17) • Peach (1 = 38) • Pear (1 = 96) • Persimmon (1 = 118) • Prune (4 = 80) • Tangerine (1 = 47)

High Glycemic Index (eat sparingly or after a workout): Banana (1 small = 90) • Grape (15 = 30) • Mango (1 = 135) • Papaya (1 small = 59) • Pineapple (1 cup = 83) • Raisin (small box = 129) • Watermelon (2 cups = 92)

Summary

Feeling hungry yet? Once you calculate your total metabolic rate and your body-fat percentage, you are ready to go. To recap, the options for creating your own food plan are:

1. Pick from the optimal-foods lists and put those foods into your meal plan.
2. Use the recipes provided to make meals, and then plug those into your meal-planning worksheet.
3. Use your own recipes. You will need to replace the unhealthful ingredients for more healthful ones. Second, you will need to calculate the calories per serving. This is done by adding the individual ingredients to get the total calories for the recipe. Divide that total by the number of servings the recipe makes. If you are unsure about serving sizes, refer to the pictures on page 145.

What goes hand-in-hand with eating nutrient-dense foods specific to the needs of your metabolism and your health? Exercise. You are probably thinking, "Ugh, now I have to exercise," "Exercising to get rid of fat takes too long," or "I run on the treadmill for an hour and a half, and I haven't lost weight." That's because there's a right way and a not-so-right way to do it. Exercising to get lean and burn fat is about working smarter, not harder. Would you be interested in a method of exercise that has been scientifically proven to change your body composition and reverse disease in less than 30 minutes a day? How about a type of exercise that causes fat burning to continue for hours or days later?

In the next chapter you will read about the most powerful method of fat burning through exercise. No gimmicks, no goofy weight-loss machines, just proven steps to cut your workout time in half and create a lean, fat-burning, and healthy body.

Get ready to transform yourself.

D
I
E

TRANSFORM

Exercise Smart and Fast

To transform means to change in appearance, form, or structure. By implementing the steps in this book, you will transform your mind, your body, and your life.

Stop! Before you read on, I want you to take a picture of yourself now . . . today. Why? Because today is a new starting point, a new beginning. It's the day you start to transform. Whether the picture shows you in a bathing suit, T-shirt and shorts, tank top, a dress, or, for the guys, your shirt off . . . just do it. Although taking the picture may make you uncomfortable, by implementing the tips and tools in this book you will transform yourself from a body you aren't satisfied with to a body that is leaner, more fit, and healthier. Having pictures of yourself before and after will be evidence of your **decision** to get healthy, lean, and fit. Having the before-and-after pictures shows that **indulging** in a variety of nutrient-dense, low-calorie foods has ignited the change in your body composition from being over-fat to having the body you want and deserve. Your before-and-after shots will give you a sense of **enjoy**ment and happiness, and enable you to see the fruits of your efforts. Finally, before-and-after pictures will show that you were able to **transform** yourself—mind and body.

Transforming is a process that requires several different states of mind. David Bliss, the retired CEO of a management-and-consulting company, describes the "states of change" a person goes through in order to transform from "now" to a place in the future. The transformation happens in three stages: your current state; the future state, which is where you want to be; and the transition state, which is the time between where you are now and where you want to be.

The Current State

Being unhappy with your body and the way you feel, along with wanting to rebuild your health, is most likely the reason you chose this book. You must believe that staying the way you are—whether you are over-fat, fatigued, or dealing with chronic health issues—is no longer an option for you. Ask yourself why you want to transform. Perhaps you're sick of seeing yourself in "cover-up" clothes because you're embarrassed about your body. Maybe you fear the future health issues you might face if you don't change. Are you modifying your lifestyle to be around longer for your children? Whatever your reason, you have to *feel* the reason—not just know it intellectually, but feel it in your heart. Once you have done this, you will set in motion the steps to improve your body composition and your health.

The Transition State

In this state, you are no longer content with prior unhealthful habits, but you are not yet where you want to be. As you travel along your journey— changing the way you eat, putting in place an exercise schedule, and improving your lifestyle—sometimes you hit bumps in the road. To keep yourself going strong, you will 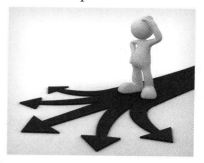 need support, motivation, reinforcement, a measurement of progress, and celebration of the small victories along the way. Let's talk about these important factors.

Support: It's OK to share your fears and struggles with your spouse, friends, and family members as you go through this process. Sometimes it's hard to open up and share because that makes you vulnerable. Look for people who are nonjudgmental, who make you laugh and boost you up when you need a lift.

Motivation: Nothing matches the feeling you have when someone pumps you up, gives you strength, and helps to provide the motivation to succeed. Look to those with whom you can exercise, cook, and share meals and recipes for constant motivation.

Reinforcement and Measurement of Progress: These go hand in hand. Change can be difficult and frustrating, but it can also be rewarding. When your body composition changes, and your weight goes down as a consequence of getting rid of the fat—that is a measurement of progress. Measuring your progress can also be done with the formulas (BMI, BMR, and your body-fat percentage). What about your health progress? An improvement in your health can be seen with new blood work, hormone profiling, or any other method of testing that was used initially to diagnose your condition. New testing also can provide a prognosis for your condition. Perhaps your inflammation markers—C-reactive protein and erythrocyte sedimentation rate (ESR)—have improved, or your fasting blood sugar and hemoglobin A1c (markers of diabetes) are back to normal. Whatever the markers were to diagnose your condition(s), retest them to monitor your progress. These measurable changes will show you that your efforts are paying off. That deserves a "great job!" Positive reinforcement is also key to keeping you from falling off the wagon.

Celebration: As you meet your short-term goals, reward yourself by doing something that makes you feel good. Perhaps you buy a new pair of shoes, a new exercise outfit, or a new iPod you can load with heart-pumpin' music. Maybe enjoy a night on the town or a quiet relaxing weekend away. Reward yourself with whatever makes you feel good, whatever keeps you motivated to get you through the transition state.

Sally D. reached a point where her health and her body composition were unsustainable. Her BMI was above 35, and her body-fat percentage was far too high. Yet a big part of her problem was her lack of confidence that she could become more fit. Following her first visit, I suggested seeing her every two weeks to monitor her progress and help her stay on track. Knowing that she was going to receive a boost, she went to work. After only two weeks on the Body Composition Diet, she had dropped weight, lost body fat, and started to feel better. "This is awesome!" I told her. That brought a smile to her face, and I followed that with a hug and a high five. I knew she was now determined to continue with her positive lifestyle changes. She had struggled with dieting in the past partly because she didn't have the positive reinforcement to keep her head in the game. Now Sally has lost 55 pounds of body fat, feels great, and is actively involved in an exercise program she enjoys.

The Future State

You must have a clear, motivating picture of the future you want to create. This ideal must be emotionally felt and owned by you; someone can't just tell you it would be good for you. What does the future look like in your mind's eye? A newly built body? Getting off medications and the reversal of your health issues? Maybe you dream of walking into your favorite store to buy that outfit you've always wanted. Or maybe you want to live a healthful life so you can be a more active parent. Whatever this future state looks like for you, you must feel it. Going through change because your spouse or family has been nagging you is not sustainable. What's *your* motivation for change? What's *your* mental finish line?

Lose the Fat, Save the Muscle—At Any Age

Weight loss has always been synonymous with size. The weight-loss industry spends zillions of dollars advertising the "get thin, lean, and sexy" mindset. Of course, in order to do this, you must buy some product or program. While being lean is important for a multitude of reasons, the goal of healthy weight management is better body composition. It's about losing fat. From today on, divorce yourself from the notion of "weight loss" and focus on *fat loss*.

You may have noticed that throughout this book I have made the distinction between weight and fat. We all think we know the difference between fat and muscle. Yet many people trying to lose surely don't act that way. In order for you to take full advantage of the exercises I am going to suggest later in this chapter, it's worth making sure that you do understand what you're working for. That's the best way to change your shape.

What Is Fat?

Fat (adipose tissue) is the body's built-in battery; its main role is to store energy. Along with providing energy, it insulates and cushions the body. Believe it or not, fat is a hormone-producing tissue. It can produce hormones like leptin (which helps to control appetite) and adiponectin (which helps to burn fat). Fat also makes estrogen—do you recall aromatase?

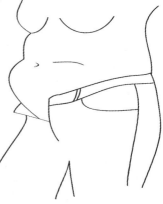

Different kinds of fat appear in different parts of the body. The visible fat just under the skin is called subcutaneous fat. While this type of fat poses no real health threat, it is the one that everyone is trying to lose. However, the invisible fat that can surround organs is called visceral fat, which is very dangerous. Visceral fat, or "belly fat," has been linked to heart disease, cancer, and diabetes. As I previously mentioned, fat of any kind, specifically the fat surrounding the organs and the fat that pushes through your belt line, is toxic. Fat not only produces hormones that alter your appetite, it's also a source of inflammation. Again, it's not the type of inflammation caused by a sprained ankle; it's the type that creates a battle zone within your immune system to wage war on your body, which could ultimately lead to chronic disease.

What Is Lean Muscle?

Muscles are the body's motors; they produce force and cause motion by contraction (shortening). Muscle tissue is biologically active and requires a lot more calories to fuel itself than fat tissue does. Therefore, the more lean muscle you have, the faster your metabolism is, which allows you to burn more calories in a day. There are two types of muscles in the body—smooth and skeletal. Smooth muscle makes up the heart and is found in the walls of organs, e.g., intestines and blood vessels. We will focus on skeletal muscle, which drives your metabolism and is a major component of body composition

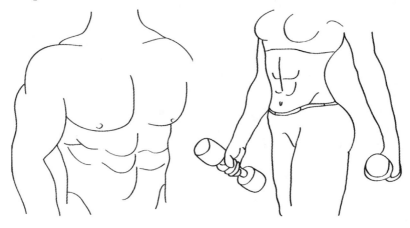

Real "dieting" is about body composition—decrease the body fat and increase the lean muscle. When people lose weight rapidly, they lose not only fat; they lose muscle. That's not healthy. I will show you how to get rid of the fat and preserve your muscle. Wouldn't it be nice if that could be accomplished without much effort? Is it possible? Yep! So much effort is put into losing fat *fast* through major restrictive diets and physically exhausting workout programs. While losing the fat is a goal, the Body Composition Diet gives you tools to *stop making the fat*. The best way to lose it is to stop making it, while you get rid of the fat you have. Again, this is done by combining highly nutritious, fat-burning foods with the right kind of exercise.

Body Types

Being over-fat is a major risk factor for our most serious diseases. A simple measurement to determine your risk for illness is your waist circumference, as well as the waist-to-hip ratio. When your waist increases in size, so does your risk. For men, a waist circumference of 40 inches or more is a red flag for cardiovascular disease and diabetes. For women, a waist circumference of 35 inches or more increases the risk for those same illnesses.

Measure your waist-to-hip ratio. You do this by measuring the circumference of your waist and the circumference of your hips (feet together). Use the lines on the diagram below as guide points for the measuring tape. Divide the waist measurement by the hip measurement to get the waist/hip ratio. Research shows that this ratio is a far better measurement for determining risk for serious disease than just the waist measurement alone. For men, any number at 1 or above is at risk; for women, any number of .8 or above is a significant risk.

The Apple Body

The apple-shaped body is one of accumulated fat in the midsection—subcutaneous fat and visceral fat—and is linked to heart disease, diabetes, gallbladder disease, high blood pressure, and stroke. This body type is more common in men, but frequently develops in post-menopausal women. Research suggests that a buildup of fat around the midsection poses a higher risk for disease than a fat buildup around the hips.

Waist-to-Hip Ratio:
Men at or above 1
Women at or above .8

This body shape is also associated with insulin resistance, type 2 diabetes, and high blood lipids like cholesterol and triglycerides.

The Pear Body

This body type has hips that are wider than the shoulders because fat is stored around on the hips and butt. This extra

weight (fat) around the hips poses less risk
for serious illnesses.

The pear body is associated with a hormone
imbalance that includes estrogen, thyroid
hormones, and the stress hormone cortisol.
Some literature suggests this body
type is associated with poor hormone
detoxification by the liver.

The Spare Tire/Muffin Top

Ah, the unwanted spare tire. This fat is noticeable when
wearing tight jeans; the fat comes up and over your belt line.
The spare tire is associated with
low-grade embarrassment, and
the desire to wear slightly bigger
clothing for camouflage. It also
puts a brake on taking your shirt
off in public.

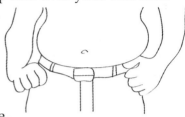

Regardless of your body type,
excessive body fat is unhealthy. Along with diabetes and
cardiovascular disease, it can also cause internal inflammation,
which can set off certain cancers. That's another reason why
using the tips and tools in this book is so important for your
health.

WARNING: You Can't Out-Train a Crappy Diet

Before we get to different exercises you might want to try, I
should make one point clear. You're fooling yourself if you
think you can out-train a diet of high-calorie, low-nutrient-
dense, processed foods. The reason for this isn't hard to find.
If you eat more calories than your body uses on a daily basis,
you're going to increase your body fat. If you continue to eat
the same unhealthful high-calorie foods, and your exercise
doesn't burn the calories you've eaten—again, you're going
to increase your body fat. For example, let's say you burn off
270 calories during 20 minutes of exercise and then reward
yourself by eating a bag of French fries that contains 420

calories. Guess what's going to happen? That's why food really is the control. When you combine exercising with eating healthful foods, you'll get a healthy body composition.

"I can't give up my wine, and I love to eat," Nicole K. tells me as she exhausts herself running on a treadmill at the gym. She was running when I walked into the gym, and was still going 45 minutes later, when I was walking out. I told her, "You can't out-train a crappy diet." Her lifestyle included eating all the wrong types of food and drinking at night to relax after a long stressful day. Her frustration was not being able to lose the fat, although she was on the treadmill an hour a day. This is a classic example of her poor diet undercutting her fat-loss efforts.

Let's say you are more mindful of what you eat. You decide to go out for dinner after a long day. You sit with your spouse, friends, or family and start the process of ordering dinner. The typical scenario at a restaurant starts with bread, washed down with some alcoholic beverage—wine or spirits. You then order a salad, thinking it's the healthful thing to do, and follow it with the main course. For many, that is pasta or a large protein meal combined with a high-calorie carbohydrate like baked or mashed potatoes. Oh, let's not forget the second glass of wine. The meal is then 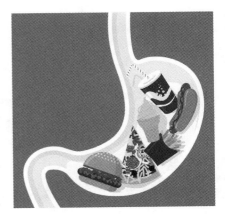 topped off with a refined, sugary dessert. Shortly after your super-calorie-charged meal, at home you change into your PJs and chill out before bed thinking to yourself, "Ugh, I ate too much." You retire to bed, fall asleep (maybe), and your body gets to work. As it digests the meal, your pancreas is working hard, spitting insulin into your blood to try to lower the incredible influx of sugar and calories from the meal. Insulin works hard to help get the now-high blood sugar to the liver and your skeletal muscles. Once they've had enough, insulin helps to store the rest of the sugar and excess calories in your fat cells. Those fat cells swell, and you get fat while you sleep.

The next morning, feeling like crap and guilty for eating last night's calories, you rationalize the big meal by thinking you can burn those calories by working out. Still not feeling super energized, you push through a full 60-minute workout in the hope that you just burned off all that you ate. However, the problem is that eating a big meal late in the evening is not just making you fatter, it's messing up your hormones. My point in illustrating this scenario is: You can't out-train a crappy diet. More specifically, eating high-calorie meals at night will make you fatter . . . guaranteed!

Prevent and Reverse Disease with Exercise

Extensive research has proven that regular exercise has a wide range of health benefits, including improved cardiovascular function, improved muscle mass, and bone health. Exercise has also been shown to help the immune system fight disease, reduce free-radical damage, reduce inflammation, regulate blood sugar, and prevent excessive body fat.

The Scandinavian Journal of Medicine and Science in Sports refers to using exercise as therapy for a wide range of disorders such as insulin resistance, type 2 diabetes, hypertension, obesity, heart disease, osteoporosis, depression, and cancer. *Circulation*, the journal of the American Heart Association, states that long-term physical exercise improves relaxation of the blood vessels through the release of nitric oxide. Nitric oxide (NO) is a chemical that "talks" to the smooth muscle in blood vessels. This relaxation allows for less restricted blood flow, thus improving conditions of the heart and reducing high blood pressure.

Can exercising improve brain function and other conditions associated with the brain? *Clinical Practice & Epidemiology in Mental Health* has found that exercising can significantly fight against depression, and that it can be used as an alternative to current medications for depression.

Additional research from the journal *Acta Biomed* shows that regular exercise has been shown to reduce visceral fat (internal belly fat), help insulin sensitivity, improve glucose and blood-pressure control, and improve blood-lipid profiles. It further goes on to say, "For these reasons, regular aerobic physical activity must be considered an essential component of the cure of type 2 diabetes."

Jack B., a retired airline pilot, handed me his blood tests after seeing his cardiologist, who told him his blood work was fine except for the high triglycerides. Sadly, Jack's doctor missed the high blood sugar and elevated hemoglobin A1c. Both screamed type 2 diabetes. Since his father had died from Alzheimer's disease, and his mother because of pancreatic cancer—both associated with blood-sugar problems—Jack was really concerned. He was also frustrated with his lack of energy and the belly fat that he could no longer stand to look at. Once he started eating the right healthful foods, the belly fat melted away, and his energy came back. Eight weeks later, I sent him out for blood work again. His results revealed normal triglycerides, his fasting sugar (blood-sugar level after sleeping) was back to normal, and the hemoglobin A1c had dramatically dropped. Eager to show his cardiologist the changes, Jack paid him a visit and showed him the blood work. His doctor's question was, "Oh, my God, how did you do this?" Jack's response: "Dr. Z's Body Composition Diet."

So now it's time for the third and final Dr. Z Rule. That's tough, right? Only three rules you have to keep in mind. Do you think you can follow them to achieve that new you?

Z Rule #3. Burst to Burn and Rebuild: High-intensity interval training creates a healthy body composition.

Long periods of endurance exercise have long been associated with burning fat. Gyms are filled with people running, oscillating, and climbing stairs for hours on end in the hope of melting off body fat. Yet, for most people, longtime exercise with moderate intensity comes up short in producing fat loss. Research is finding that high-intensity exercise done in short periods 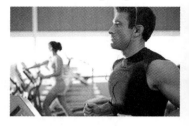 improves fat oxidation (burning) better than high-volume training (endurance).

Endurance training involves exercising at a steady pace for 20 minutes or longer. This type of exercise is usually performed at a gym or at home on machines like a treadmill, elliptical machine, stair-climber, or any other machine found in the cardio section of the gym. Long-distance running and bike riding are also considered endurance exercises. Hardcore endurance junkies engage in major long-distance cycling and triathlons. Endurance training has always been associated with heart health. This form of aerobic exercise can strengthen the heart, improve circulation—allowing more oxygen to get into the body—and improve skeletal muscle strength.

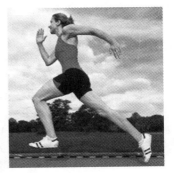

High-intensity interval training (HIIT) typically involves all-out intensity for a short period, followed by periods of low-intensity exercise or rest. A great example of this is sprinting—explosive movement for a short time, followed by a walk or rest. The most used program in the research is the Wingate protocol, which involves high-intensity sprinting for 30 seconds with hard resistance. This is done four to six times separated by four-minute rest periods, performed three times a week for two to six weeks. Although this routine may seem simple, it is very effective. Other researchers have created modified high-intensity protocols, all of which were very effective at getting rid of fat and greatly improving metabolism. I have included a very effective high-intensity interval training routine that takes little time and has a major impact. You won't believe the results.

The Research Behind High-Intensity Interval Training

In the *Journal of Applied Physiology*, researchers found that seven sessions of high-intensity interval training over a two-week period improved whole-body-fat oxidation (burning) as well as the capacity for skeletal muscles to burn fat. Studies from different sources all show that high-intensity interval training is a very effective way to reduce not only subcutaneous fat, but also visceral fat (surrounding organs). According to the journal *Metabolic Syndrome and Related Disorders*, short-term, high-intensity aerobic exercise reduced visceral fat in overweight adults. Remember, visceral fat is the kind that has been related to many chronic diseases, like heart disease, diabetes, and cancer.

An article written in *Cancer Research* states that exercise by women whose percentage of body fat decreased by two percent resulted in a significant decrease in estrogen. Why is this important for women and men? Because body fat creates estrogen, which is a major spark for cancers of the breast, endometrium, and ovaries, as well as the prostate in men.

Research found in the *British Medical Journal* and *Acta Oncologica* revealed high-intensity exercising improved cardiopulmonary (heart and lung) function, muscle strength, aerobic capacity, and emotional well-being, as well as reduced fatigue in those being treated with chemotherapy for advanced cancers. A study published in *Physiological Reviews* found intense exercising for short periods was shown to increase natural killer cell—a type of white blood cell that kills cancer—activity for hours after exercising. Perfect. High-intensity interval training . . . a self-induced cancer treatment.

For heart disease, HIIT is also superior to aerobic exercise with moderate intensity. Data found in *Australian Family Physician* and *Circulation* states that high-intensity interval training reduced LDL cholesterol, while increasing HDL cholesterol. HIIT was also found to improve endothelial function, blood pressure, left ventricular function and glucose regulation. High-intensity training was found to be safe for those with pre-existing heart disease, and those who had already suffered a heart attack. Furthermore, *Australian Family Physician* found that periods of exercising with intensity were beneficial for those with stable angina, as well as post-cardiac stenting and after coronary-artery grafting.

In the journal *Metabolism*, researchers found that high-intensity training was far better than exercising at a constant pace with moderate intensity for getting rid of subcutaneous fat. High-intensity training, according to the *International Journal of Obesity*, is a very efficient way not only to burn fat, but to reduce depositing it in the body and to improve metabolism.

High-intensity interval training is also the exercise of choice to regulate insulin, growth hormone, and glucagon. Through studies found in the *European Journal of Applied Physiology*, the *Journal of Applied Physiology*, and the *Journal of Nutrition and Metabolism*, exercising with intensity increased the release of growth hormone and helped to balance insulin and glucagon. If you remember, insulin stores fat and glucagon burns fat. Growth hormone, released after exercising, helps to build muscle and, like glucagon, causes the body to burn fat for fuel.

Exercise Smarter, Not Harder!

You may have seen different high-intensity workouts like the Wingate protocol, but I'd like to share an effective one I use, which requires only 20 minutes per session.

As an example, I will describe my high-intensity aerobic training on an at-home treadmill that I use during inclement and cold weather. If you have a treadmill, it's time to remove the boxes and jackets thrown on it and give it a dusting. After turning on the machine, I start with a low-intensity (level two) walk for two minutes. While walking, I'm getting a feel for the machine, and I'm warming up my legs. After those two minutes, I increase the speed on the treadmill to a moderate intensity (level four or five). This takes me from a nice-paced walk to a super-fast walk or slow jog. I continue this pace for one minute. Then it's time for the high-energy, high-intensity run. I increase the speed on the machine to a level eight or nine. I run at top speed for one minute. You don't think a minute is long, but at an all-out effort, it is. My heart rate elevates, and my muscles feel as though they are starting to get pumped. Once the minute is up, I quickly slow down back to the low intensity I started with for two minutes. Following the two minutes, I speed back up to a level four or five of moderate intensity for one minute, then again all-out exertion at level eight or nine for one minute, followed by throttling down to the two-minute low intensity.

Note: For many, going all-out for one minute is tough. So maybe just start off at 30 seconds. As you get more conditioned, go to 45 seconds and then perhaps 60 seconds. Your high-intensity set may be only 30 seconds; that's OK. Everybody is different. You need to find the level that challenges you enough to burn the fat and increase your metabolism.

I repeat this sequence five times, and then cool down with a three-to-five-minute walk of low intensity on the treadmill, or just walk around for a bit until I'm somewhat rested. This exercise sequence will make you feel as if you've worked out. Following this sweat session, I know that I'm burning fat for hours to come. This sequence takes roughly 20 minutes; the cool-down is another five. Inside, I usually use a treadmill or a stationary bike. I use a road bike when I'm training outside.

When you're just beginning to exercise with intensity, start by walking, riding, or moving on a treadmill, elliptical machine, or stair-climber for four to five minutes just to get your head into it. Once you are used to a workout that fits you, you may not need to spend time doing this. Once you condition yourself, start the two-minute low-level intensity as soon as you begin. Your ability to exercise with intensity is probably different from mine.

Your "level nine" is based on your fitness level. Don't stress by comparing yourself to others, or get frustrated because you think you should train like an iron man. Once you start your own high-intensity interval-training program, you can test your initial abilities and change them as you progress.

If you are a runner, sprint on the hills for the high-intensity set, or just sprint on a level surface if you're not near a hill. If you're a cyclist, cycle up a steep hill with intensity, or if you are on a stationary bike, you can increase its resistance, or stand up to increase the intensity. Whatever the sport, figure out how to exercise with periods of low intensity, moderate intensity, and then high intensity.

Second, make sure that you are able to do this physically. Make sure you have no health issues to prevent you from exercising, or any health issues that may be exacerbated by this workout. Before beginning, you may want to consult an

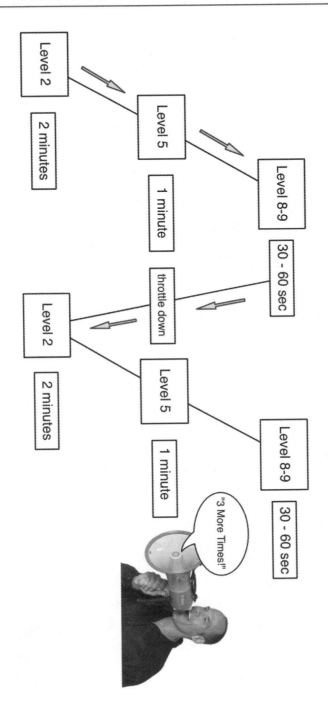

experienced healthcare practitioner—one that understands how exercising benefits the body. If you are not used to exercising, you may want to adopt a low-intensity exercise program first and then increase the frequency and duration of the exercise as you become able to train with more intensity.

"I love this!" Jen B. remarked after implementing high-intensity interval training into her workout routine. Jen had been bored with her current routine. She signed up for many different exercise classes at the gym and spent lots of time there keeping in shape. Being a mother of two, and in the midst of writing a novel, she was looking for a more effective way to stay toned. Once I introduced her to the concept of high intensity, she became very excited, not just because of a new workout, but because she could reduce her workout time by half, allowing more time for her family and her passion for writing.

Don't worry if you are not a sprinter. High-intensity interval training can be performed on a bike, treadmill, oscillating machine, any other exercise machine, or just on your own two feet. You can create a high-intensity interval-training program using TRX, kettle bells, or boot-camp training. What's the right type of high-intensity interval-training exercise for you? That's hard to say, because I don't know your abilities, disabilities, access to exercise equipment, environmental restrictions, and/or health issues that may hinder your ability to exercise with intensity. Pick any aerobic exercise as long as you can increase your intensity in intervals. The great news is that high-intensity interval training involves less learning and less time. You don't have to spend all day at the gym, or exercise for hours on end until you're exhausted. Twenty minutes of high intensity allows for maximum fat burning!

When Is the Best Time to Exercise?

I realize everyone has a busy schedule, so finding time to exercise can sometimes be challenging. The good news is that you require only about 20 minutes of high-

intensity interval training to burn fat and maintain your muscle. The answer to the question "When is the best time to exercise?" is more variable. Here's the story: Whether it's high-intensity interval training, weight training, or some other form of resistance exercise, you should not do it on an empty stomach. A safe time to exercise is about one to four hours after eating a small meal. Why? The delay allows the stomach to empty. By that time your blood sugar has risen and is stored in the muscle as glycogen.

Pre-exercise eating is very important. Let's say you get up, swill down a cup of coffee, and head off to the gym. Because you haven't eaten overnight, your blood sugar is low. If you exercise with no fuel, your body reaches for your muscle sugar first. Then you deplete your liver sugar. After that, your body depends on hormones to break down muscle in order to provide you with the blood sugar for continued exercise. This is not what you want to do. Remember body composition? Lose the fat, build the muscle. Exercising without fuel can cause you to lose valuable muscle.

It's worth going back over what cortisol does inside your body. As you remember, cortisol is a hormone released from the adrenal glands during times of stress. Cortisol is an anti-inflammatory hormone, which means it helps to control any allergic responses, as well as helping to regulate blood sugar. However, when your blood sugar is low, cortisol can have an adverse effect. The brain's only fuel source is glucose, so when blood sugars are low, cortisol breaks down muscle, turning it into glucose for the brain's survival. Muscles require sugar in order for them to perform during exercising. If you don't eat before exercising, you may not have the right amount of fuel to work out. Cortisol will break down the muscle, and at the same time it will maintain the fat, because the brain can't use fat as a fuel source.

To prevent this from happening, eat a small amount of protein with some form of complex carbohydrate a minimum of 60 to 90 minutes before you exercise. This should provide the muscles with fuel and block muscle breakdown. If you eat too much before exercising, you may be nauseated. That's because your body is trying to digest the food and at the same time manage your muscles and heart during the activity. So wait at least one hour after eating before you exercise.

What time of day is best for exercise? Cortisol follows a circadian rhythm; it is highest in the morning and lowest at night. Some research studies have found that exercising in the afternoon is best; others advise exercising in the morning. My opinion is to make sure you eat before you work out . . . period. Cortisol will rise when you haven't eaten, and it is also highest after exercising. In addition, post-exercise eating is very important. You need to refuel your muscles to prevent cortisol from breaking them down.

Keep in mind a couple of guidelines. Always exercise 60 to 90 minutes after eating to maintain your blood sugar. Choose the time of day that works for you to get in weight training and high-intensity interval training, and definitely eat a serving of protein with a serving of carbs after the workout to prevent the effects of cortisol, and to load your muscles with glycogen (muscle sugar) again.

Let me point out again that you can't out-train a crappy diet. If you are exercising until exhaustion thinking that you can burn off the pizza from the night before, you're sadly mistaken. Dieting first, coupled with high-intensity interval training, is the best strategy to burn fat and get lean. Since lean muscle eats excessive calories and burns fat, creating it or having more of it has a big impact on a healthy body composition. Building a lean and muscular body is best done with high-intensity training and resistance training (strength training) that you can do right at home or at your local gym.

Not Seeing the Results?

There are many reasons why people can't get rid of fat— from not knowing what to eat, how much to eat and when, to uncontrollable, emotional eating. There also can be undiscovered physical reasons behind failed attempts in the fat-loss arena. Those physical or biological issues not only prevent fat loss, they can lead to discouragement. Eventually, you may give up on "diets," thinking they don't work. Let's not forget the frustrations about exercise; too much or too little can prevent you from achieving better body composition. If you are running into obstacles along your fat-loss journey, it will help to know the obvious, and not so obvious, reasons why your body composition is not changing.

Just wing it. What you eat, combined with your activity level, determines how well your metabolism functions. Your unique metabolism is based on your body's systems, e.g., heart and circulation, digestion, and muscular structure. Your caloric calculation is meant to stop the production of fat, burn existing fat, and maintain lean muscle. If you are overeating or undereating, you either will be making fat or holding on to it. Major calorie restriction also causes the release of the hormone ghrelin, which increases appetite and eventually causes overeating.

They're not my type. What you eat is just as important as how much. Eating 1,300 calories of pizza, fast food, soda, and ice cream is completely different from eating 1,300 calories of healthful proteins, greens, starchy vegetables, nuts, seeds, and fruit. Food is information. It not only gives us energy; it provides the nutrients that keep us free of disease. High-calorie processed foods not only will create disease; they will increase insulin, the hormone that makes you fat.

Exercise aversion. "It takes too long." "It's too much effort." These are thoughts that may prevent you from getting started. Good news! Exercising to burn fat, rebuild from disease, and prevent disease takes only 20 to 30 minutes a day, or every other day. Spending a day at the gym is a waste of time and actually may hinder your fat-loss goals. Exercising with intensity rather than duration is the best way to get rid of flab on the abs. On the other hand, deciding to blow off exercise will definitely slow down your fat-loss goals. Remember not to overtrain or push too hard right out of the gate. You want to build up gradually so you stay the course, rather than hitting it hard, which might leave you sore and discouraged.

Bad moon rising. When the sun goes down and the moon comes out, that is a sign to reduce your food consumption. You should eat during the day when you're active, not when you're getting ready for bed. If you eat most of your calories at night, you are definitely storing fat and increasing internal inflammation. Food is meant to be eaten and burned during the day, not eaten and stored as fat while you sleep. If you have to eat in the evening, choose green and rainbow-colored vegetables with a small piece of protein. This will have little effect on the hormones that store fat while you're snoozing.

Taking the wrong approach. How you approach the challenge of changing your body composition and your health starts with a decision. For some, the "all-or-nothing" approach works; others prefer setting small, realistic goals. Perhaps start with a walk every day until you are ready to engage in more strenuous exercise. Likewise, substitute coconut-milk ice cream for regular ice cream. Making small changes will ease the transition into a regular pattern of more healthful eating and exercising, which will serve not only your body composition, but also your long-term health.

Sleep issues. Sleep is important, not just for overall health, but also to get rid of the bulge. Poor sleep patterns create simple-sugar cravings during the day, which is counterproductive for fat-loss goals. Poor sleep can be caused by many things, including life stressors, progesterone deficiency, eating late at night, and alcohol consumption. Make it a priority to discover and resolve the culprit behind your sleep problems. Read about the benefits of good sleep on page 103 in "Dr. Z's Indulging Tips and Tools."

Stress. Stress increases cortisol, which causes fat to be stored in the belly. Stress also can cause overeating. When we are burned out from a stressful day, we tend to overeat refined, high-calorie foods, the ones that create that unwanted muffin top. These simple-sugar foods relax us temporarily, causing a boost of serotonin, which makes us feel good in the short term. Identify your stressors and find a way to deal with them that won't make you sick or fat. Refer to the list of "low points" and how to deal with them that you created in the "Decide" chapter.

Self-defense. A strong connection exists between obesity and sexual abuse or other serious emotional trauma. It is natural to protect yourself when you have been traumatized or violated in any way. Subconsciously, being over-fat can make you less attractive to others. It also may shut down sexuality and keep your libido in check. If you have been traumatized in any way, seek help from a counselor, one who specializes in recovering from sexual abuse and post-traumatic stress.

Don't give up on yourself. If you miss exercise one day, or eat something you shouldn't, don't stress. Just dust yourself off and get back on track the next day. Having a bad day does not mean you "can't do this" or "all is lost." Reconnect with the real reason you have chosen to change your lifestyle—the emotionally felt reason. That will guide you back to a pattern of consistent behavior and help you to avoid feeling guilty when you have an off day. Remember, if you give up on your body, it will give up on you.

Burn Away That Fat

For best results, combine high-intensity interval training with weight training. First make sure you are physically able to train with weights. If so, you will find that weight training or resistance training can play a key role in changing your body composition. That's because the faster your metabolism, the more fat you will burn off. Lean muscle is the fountain of youth. Research is showing that resistance training with weights has numerous benefits, such as regulating blood sugar and insulin, slowing down the aging process of our cells, and improving strength and endurance. What is resistance training? Resistance training (strength training) is a form of exercise that causes your muscles to push against some force, or resistance. Probably the best example of this form of exercise is weight lifting. Using weights to lift or machines to push against increases the strength and size of the muscles involved. Other examples of strength training are resistance bands, swimming machines, kettle bells, TRX, and the Bowflex machines.

In the *Journal of Applied Physiology*, researchers found that resistance exercise with weights improved body composition by burning fat throughout the body, specifically abdominal (belly) fat. This research supports the findings of many other research articles about resistance training with weights.

Coupling high-intensity interval training with aerobic exercise or with weight or resistance exercise is the ultimate way to improve your body composition and rebuild your body.

Developing a resistance-training protocol for yourself depends on your abilities. When you exercise with resistance or weight, you do it based on your fitness level. At the start, pick weights that allow you to do 10 to 12 repetitions. As you get stronger, you can increase the amount of weight you are using per exercise.

Here's an example of high-intensity interval training with resistance exercise using weights: a shoulder exercise like a seated dumbbell press. I will usually start with 50 pounds as my first set. I press the dumbbells 10 to 12 reps, a comfortable range and weight for me. Once I'm done with that set, I look at my watch and time the next minute or minute and a half. I then grab the 60s and press them for eight reps. Again, I wait a minute or minute and a half, then press the 70-pound dumbbells for a set of six, then the fourth set at 80 pounds for four reps. I'm using these weights because I can. There is no contest here; I'm lifting those weights based on my ability. You may use 10 or 15 pounds. Make sure you are comfortable with the weights you use so you don't hurt yourself. Try working out with someone who can spot you. A trainer can also guide you and spot you.

For my last set, I drop the weight back down to 50 pounds and go back to the 10 to 12 reps for maximum intensity. This is the high-intensity interval training set. Once completed, I cool down for a couple of minutes.

Ready for the Stage

I'm an amateur figure competitor and a personal trainer. I met Dr. Z in graduate school. We spent much time discussing diet-and-exercise trends during class breaks. Dr. Z told me about the Body Composition Diet in *Rebuild*, and I decided to give it a trial run. I used the diet in my contest prep this season. My training consists of high-intensity interval cardio training; I'll do sprints on an elliptical or stationary bike on my cardio days for about 25 minutes, usually four times a week. I also hit the weight room, working each body part twice a week. I lift heavy in order to build muscle and shape my physique. Several times a day, I eat low-calorie, nutritionally dense foods with carbohydrates focused more during the daytime hours and no carbs after 6 p.m.

The change in my body was pretty dramatic and very fast. After about two weeks of exercising and eating this way, my body started to lean out and take shape. I've been really happy with my results and recommend Dr. Z's diet to all of my personal training and competitor clients.

—Linda S.

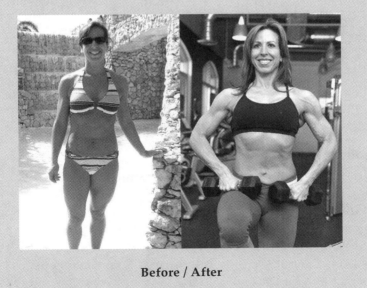

Before / After

Seated Dumbbell Press

Sit on a stable bench or chair with your feet firmly planted on the ground and your back against the back of the chair. Lift the weights up to the starting position seen in the picture.

If the weights are heavier than you can lift straight up to your shoulders, place them on your knees and use your legs to assist lifting them.

From the starting position, push the weights while rotating them to the finished position. Once completed, slowly lower the dumbbells to the starting position.

Repeat for desired number of reps.

Seated Dumbbell Press			
Weight	Repetitions	Time Between Sets	HIIT Level
50 lbs.	10-12	1 Minute	Low – 5
70 lbs.	8	1 Minute	Medium – 6
80 lbs.	6	1 Minute	Medium – 8
90 lbs.	4	1 Minute	High - 9
50 lbs.	10-12	Last Minute	HIIT Level

Standing Barbell Curl

This is a classic for building and toning your biceps. Stand firmly on the ground.

Grab a barbell with your hands a little wider than shoulder width, palms facing out.

Slowly curl the weight up to the finished position. Do not swing while lifting. Feel the biceps contract as you lift.

Lower slowly to the starting position.

Repeat for the desired reps.

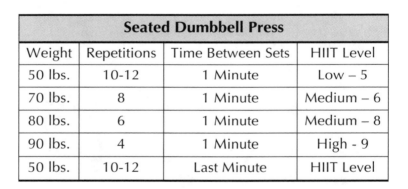

Standing Barbell Curl			
Weight	Repetitions	Time Between Sets	HIIT Level
50 lbs.	10-12	1 Minute	Low – 5
70 lbs.	8	1 Minute	Medium – 6
80 lbs.	6	1 Minute	Medium – 8
90 lbs.	4	1 Minute	High - 9
50 lbs.	10-12	Last Minute	HIIT Level

In the following chapter, I have created charts for you to keep track of your workout schedule, including upper-body exercises and lower-body exercises. I'm sure I have not included all the exercises associated with each body part; therefore, you should develop a workout program that works for you. There are many ways you can build on this program, such as using a trainer or searching online for specific types of exercise.

Exercise Schedule

My exercise schedule is illustrated in the charts below. I alternate resistance with high-intensity interval-training aerobic exercises. Allowing yourself sufficient recovery time is just as important as the training, so sometimes I take one or two days off during the week for recovery time. After the recovery, start where you left off. If your last training was 20 minutes of aerobic exercise, start with either upper- or lower-body weight training. If you ended with weights before the recovery time, start with 20 minutes of aerobics.

Monday	Tuesday	Wednesday	Thursday	Friday	Saturday	Sunday
Upper-Body Weights	20 Minutes HIIT Aerobics	Lower-Body Weights	20 Minutes HIIT Aerobics	Upper-Body Weights	20 Minutes HIIT Aerobics or Off Day	Off Day

Monday	Tuesday	Wednesday	Thursday	Friday	Saturday	Sunday
Lower-Body Weights	20 Minutes HIIT Aerobics	Upper-Body Weights	20 Minutes HIIT Aerobics	Lower-Body Weights	20 Minutes HIIT Aerobics or Off Day	Off Day

If you train using some other form of anaerobic exercise, like kettle bells, cable machines, body-weight training, sand bags, etc., create a program that encompasses multiple sets with increasing difficulty, then a high-intensity set at the end. Remember: figure out what weights and exercises you can do based on your ability. Then exercise. If you are already training for endurance, ramp up the fat-burning and muscle-building by adding two to three days of high-intensity interval training with weights. This will increase not only your strength, but also your VO_2 max, which is needed for long-endurance training. VO_2 max is a measurement of how well the body uses oxygen during exercise; it is used to determine how fit you are.

High-intensity interval training (HIIT) will also help you to reverse chronic illness, as well as to improve your energy levels and metabolism. It should also be enjoyable! By incorporating HIIT, you will begin to enjoy exercising without regret, frustration, or resentment. As you see the fat melt away and you get leaner, you will notice you reach for your sneakers instead of junk foods loaded with salt, fat, and sugar.

High-intensity interval training is mandatory in your efforts to create your ultimate body composition. When it comes to shaping your body and burning fat, there is no better way to "build and burn" than strength training with weights. Don't worry, weight training is not just for football players and body builders. Weight training has been shown to tone and build muscle, regulate your blood sugar, and burn fat. Lean muscles are like a sexy fat furnace. Once you tone and build them, you are able to burn fat long after the exercising has been completed. You may be thinking, "Wait, I don't belong to a gym," or "I'm not comfortable going to the gym." That's OK. The first ten exercises I'm going to show you can be done at home. Because I don't recommend lifting bags of cement, or throwing yourself over the back of your foot board on your bed, you will need a few items for doing these exercises at home. You may want to purchase some hand weights that you can manage. Buying a single bench that can be used for many exercises is a good idea. Last, you may want to get a yoga mat so the exercises that require you to lie or kneel on the ground aren't uncomfortable.

Here are my thoughts regarding strength training. I think just the words "strength training" and "weight lifting" can be intimidating to some. I get it. Images of climbing onto big machines, or trying to push massive plates of steel, can be nerve-wracking. So, don't do that. Leave the giant plates of steel to the people who body build and strength train for competition and sports. Strength training with weights can be done at any age, physical condition, or gender. Weights can range from one pound to hundreds of pounds, just as resistance training with machines can be simple or complex, depending on your body-composition goals. Always pick a form of exercise that makes you comfortable. I can tell you this: training with weights is one of best ways to get rid of fat, tone and build your muscles, and regain your health.

So, why aren't you doing some kind of strength training? Perhaps you're not sure what to do, or you're confused on how to get started. Maybe you haven't realized that strength training is a superior way to burn fat and build the body you've always wanted. Last, you may think you will get big and bulky if you start on a weight-training program. This is actually far from reality. Forget those images of over-muscled body builders. You just want to get toned and in shape. Getting started on an exercise program is not complicated, and there are many options. You can exercise at home or at a gym; this is entirely your choice. Perhaps you don't want to drive to the gym, because you don't like the gym scene, or it takes too long to get there. Can you still lose fat and get toned at home? Yes! The following exercises can be done at home or the gym. When designing your own personal workout schedule, look at the weekly schedule that I include to get a game plan started. Maybe you start with high-intensity training a few days a week and then do a few days of strength training. I have provided a schedule that may work for you. But there is no right or wrong here. You just need to choose what works for you.

You can find lots of exercises to tone and build your muscles, but I think there are 10 strength-training exercises that you can start with at home. I call these the top 10 "build and burn" exercises.

Dr. Z's Top 10 Build-and-Burn Exercises

NUMBER ONE
Push-Up

Push-ups build both muscle and strength in the upper body, including the chest, arms, and shoulders, and they don't require machines or weights to perform. Push-ups look easy, but for some, they pose a challenge. As with any exercise, there is a technique to performing them correctly. Poor push-up technique can cause injury to your low back and shoulders.

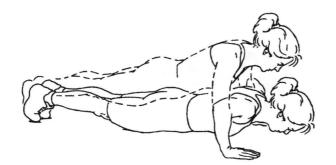

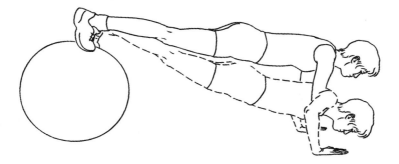

The Technique

Get into the push-up position with your elbows in a locked position.

Place your hands slightly wider than shoulder width. Keep your abs and butt (glutes) tight to avoid too much extension in your low back. Keep your head and neck in a straight line with your body. Don't look forward; keep facing down.

Lower yourself by bending your elbows until your chest almost touches the floor. Now push yourself back up to the starting position.

This exercise can also be done with a stabilization ball or yoga ball. This may be slightly more difficult because your feet are up, and you have more weight coming through your chest and arms.

Use the same technique here regarding hand placement and head and neck position, and tighten up those abs and glutes.

Repeat for the desired number of reps.

Dr. Z says . . . *"For a more challenging push-up, contract your abs and tighten your core by pulling your belly button toward your spine. While you tighten your abs, inhale as you lower yourself, and exhale as you push up off the floor."*

NUMBER TWO
One-Arm Dumbbell Row

The one-arm dumbbell row is an excellent exercise to strengthen, tone, and build your lats—the muscles that give the V-shape to your back. It also works the mid-back and rear shoulders. The picture shows the position of the dumbbell perpendicular to the bench. You can also position the weight and your hand to be parallel with the bench.

The Technique

Position yourself on the right side of the bench with your left knee and hand resting on the bench.

Pick up the dumbbell with your right hand while securing the right foot on the ground. Now, pull your shoulder blade back while keeping your arm straight. This becomes the starting position.

Pull the dumbbell up to your side until it just about makes contact with your ribs. Lower the weight until the arm is fully extended and the shoulder is stretched downward.

Repeat for desired number of reps, then repeat on the other side.

Dr. Z says . . . *"Another way to hold the weight is with the palm of your hand facing your torso. This may be more comfortable and will prevent you from brushing the weights against your side."*

NUMBER THREE
Seated Dumbbell Press

One basic shoulder exercise stands above the rest—the seated dumbbell press. Strong and shaped shoulders not only look good in a dress, suit, or on the beach; strong delts (shoulders) will give you a strong competitive edge in sports and assist in other forms of training.

The Technique

Sit on a stable bench or chair with your feet firmly planted on the ground and your back against the back of the chair. Lift the weights up to the starting position seen in the picture. If the weights are heavier than you can lift straight up to your shoulders, place them on your knees, and use your legs to assist in lifting them.

From the starting position, push the weights while rotating them to the finished position. Once completed, slowly lower the dumbbells to the starting position.

Repeat for desired number of reps.

Dr. Z says . . . *"The shoulder contains three joints surrounded by small muscles that can be injured with improper form, so don't get sloppy."*

NUMBER FOUR
Standing Dumbbell Curl

The upper arm, or biceps, is the most famous muscle(s) in the body. When I ask you to "make a muscle," what's the first muscle you think of? The biceps. The best exercise to build and shape the biceps is the standing dumbbell curl.

The Technique

Grab two dumbbells and hold them down at your sides with the palms of your hands facing your body.

Start the movement with the palm facing the body, and when the dumbbell clears your side, begin to rotate it so at the end of the movement, your palm is facing up.

As you lift the weight, feel the biceps contract all the way to the top. Now, slowly lower the weight, again with your palm facing up. When you reach the body, the dumbbell and your palm should be facing your body.

Then curl with the other arm. Repeat for desired number of reps.

Dr. Z says . . . *"Try not to cheat by swinging your body or swinging your arm through the movement. Stand still while you curl."*

NUMBER FIVE
Triceps Kickback

The triceps are made up of three heads: the long, lateral, and medial head. The lateral head is the part of the triceps that is really visible, when you extend the arm. The kickback is excellent for isolating the triceps, and it will help prevent the back of your arm from jiggling when saying good-bye.

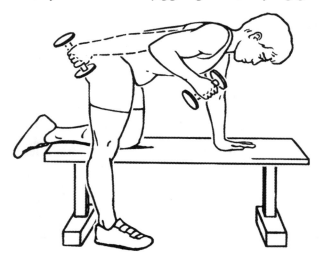

The Technique

Kneel over your bench while supporting your body with one arm. With your left knee down, and your left hand and arm supporting you, grab a dumbbell with the right hand.

Now, position your upper arm parallel to the floor. Extend the arm by contracting the triceps, until the arm is straight. Return your arm and repeat the movement.

Repeat for the desired number of reps, and then change arms.

Dr. Z says . . . *"Make sure your elbow is positioned at your side, high enough to get the full movement. To prevent poor range of motion here, have your elbow slightly higher than your shoulder. Now kick back . . . you should feel it."*

NUMBER SIX
Dumbbell Squat

The squat is a superb exercise that not only targets the upper thighs (quads) and the buttocks (glutes), it works the whole body. The major bonus with this exercise is that it not only burns a lot of calories, it also burns fat. Second, squats can improve your overall strength, your endurance and balance, and your flexibility.

The Technique
Stand with dumbbells to your sides.

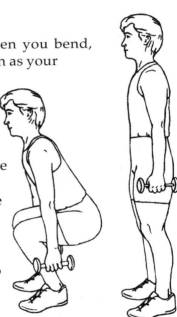

Slightly point your feet out so when you bend, your knees are facing the same direction as your feet.

Bend your knees forward while allowing your hips to bend back behind. As you lower yourself, keep your back as straight as you can and, again, your knees pointed in the same direction as your feet.

Lower yourself until your thighs are just parallel to the floor. Now, push up and extend your knees until your legs are straight.

Through the full movement, keep your head straight, back straight, and chest high. Also keep your feet firmly planted on the floor.

Repeat for the desired number of reps.

Dr. Z says . . ."*There really is no other single exercise that can improve strength, flexibility, coordination, and bone-density health than the squat. Regarding technique, it's important to stay upright. There is a tendency to lean forward here, so shift your shin bones forward and keep your heels down.*"

NUMBER SEVEN

Lunge

The lunge is really just a large step. Try taking a large step, then push yourself back up to the standing position. You will get a sense of which muscles are working and which ones will get toned with this exercise. Lunges are the quintessential quad, hamstring, and glute exercise; they are also excellent for your core.

The Technique

Stand with the dumbbells to your sides. Now, lunge forward with the first leg. As you lunge, land on your heel, then your forefoot. Once you are stable on your foot, lower your body by bending at the knee and the hip until the rear knee almost touches the ground.

Return to the original standing position by forcibly pushing back with the forward leg. Repeat the lunge with the opposite leg.

Dr. Z says . . . *"Keep your torso straight and your abs in as you push through your foot back to the starting position."*

NUMBER EIGHT
High-Knee Step Up

We all want toned and well-shaped glutes (the muscles that form the buttocks) and hamstrings (the muscles on the back of the leg). You can improve the shape of your back end by the right diet, high-intensity training, and resistance training. For keeping fat off your seat, and having shapely hams, the high-knee step up is a great exercise.

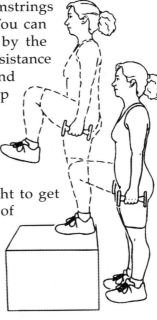

The Technique

Stand with your feet parallel about hip-width apart while holding dumbbells in your hands. Start with a light weight to get a feel for the movement and the level of difficulty.

Now, step to place your right foot on a platform, placing your foot firmly on the platform while keeping good posture. Now, push off with your left foot to raise your body onto the platform. As you come up onto the platform, continue to raise that left knee higher than the left hip, and then place that foot back down next to the right one.

On the downward phase, step backward with the left foot and place it on the ground in its starting position. Let your body lean slightly forward during the step back to create balance. Now follow with the right foot, putting it down next to the left.

Repeat these steps for the opposite side, and repeat for desired number of reps.

Dr. Z says . . . *"Try to avoid moving your foot and ankle (swaying in or out), because this will make you lose your balance. Don't make it too easy. Using a box or platform that's only a few inches tall won't challenge your hamstrings and glutes."*

NUMBER NINE
Dumbbell Calf Raise

Nothing stands out on your legs like muscular calves. The calves are tough to build because they are in constant use all day, keeping us standing and moving. The muscles that make up the calves are the soleus and the gastrocnemius muscles. They need more than just walking to get shapely and muscular. The calf raise is "the" exercise to build buff calves. The calf raise can be done multiple ways. Here is one exercise using dumbbells.

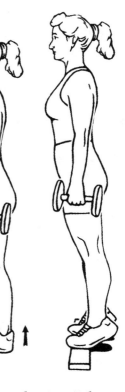

The Technique

You're going to need a small board like a 2x4 to do this exercise. Grab your dumbbells and put the balls of your feet on a stable wooden board. Your heels should be touching the floor. This is your starting position.

Point your toes straight ahead, and raise your heels off the floor by contracting the calves. As with all exercises, exhale through the movement. At the top of the contraction, hold for a second or two.

Lower yourself to the starting position. Repeat for desired number of reps.

Option 2: To provide more stability, use one dumbbell at a time. Hold a dumbbell in your right hand as you exercise the right calf. You can lean against a wall or post with the left hand for stability. Then switch hands and do the left side.

Dr. Z says . . . *"If you find the 2x4 too wobbly, or it's flipping on you, get a step platform at a gym equipment store or online. This will definitely give you stability on your toes."*

NUMBER TEN
Crunch

You can have a toned and flat stomach or a six-pack if you choose. There are two things to remember here: you have to exercise and train your abs and, most importantly, get rid of the fat overlying the muscle. The good news for you is, by following the guidelines in the Body Composition Diet, you can definitely have a toned midsection. A great exercise to start building your abs is the crunch.

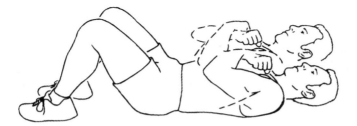

The Technique

To do a perfect crunch, lie down on the floor on your back and bend your knees. Place your hands across your chest, not behind your neck or head. By putting your hands behind your head, you tend to pull your head and neck forward, which will do your abs no good, and you may hurt your neck.

While pulling your belly button back and keeping your back flat against the floor, contract your abs, bringing your shoulders about three to five inches off the floor. Exhale while you come up, and keep your feet on the floor.

At the top of the movement, hold for a few seconds and then slowly lower yourself back down. Start again.

> **Dr. Z says . . .** *"Exhale while you come up, and squeeze those abs. See if you can do 15 to 20 reps for four to five sets."*

In the next chapter, there are other exercises you can do to build and shape your body. If you belong to a fitness facility or gym, or you are thinking of joining one, choose from these exercises to build and tone your upper and lower body and burn fat.

Transform Summary

I have added this quick checklist so you can set up the different parts of your exercise program at a glance.

First, eat a serving of protein and complex carbs roughly 90 minutes before your workout. If you don't get your blood sugar up and glycogen stored in your muscles, your body will release cortisol, which breaks down muscles to produce fuel for the brain. Second, eat protein, complex carbs, and some fruit after the workout to help quickly refuel the muscles with glycogen.

High-intensity interval training involves starting at a slow pace for two minutes, speeding up the exercise to a moderate level for one minute, and going all-out for one minute. After this high-intensity set, throttle down and start the process again at a slow pace for two minutes, speed up to a moderate pace for one minute, and, again, exercise with maximum effort for one minute. Following the high-intensity set, throttle back down to the slow level. Do this routine five times for a total of 20 minutes.

Every other day, do the same high-intensity program with weights. On one day train the upper body, the next day the lower body. Take off a day or two to recover. Without recovery time, you may be prone to aches, pain, sprains, and strains— so let the body heal. During this healing time, make sure you eat very clean foods, including protein, complex carbs, fats, vegetables, and low-sugar fruits loaded with antioxidants (blueberries, blackberries, and strawberries).

By incorporating high-intensity training into your lifestyle, you will experience an incredible change in your body composition. Exercise will help to prevent and resolve chronic health issues, which is the true prize. I hope your transformation creates changes in all aspects of your life— mind, body, and spirit.

For Serious Exercise

You are probably hungry for more build-and-burn exercises after reading through the Top 10. On pages 199 and 200, I've provided charts you can use to pick exercises to incorporate into your strength training. You can copy these pages and use them to record the exercises you choose and the weights you use.

Monday	Tuesday	Wednesday	Thursday	Friday	Saturday	Sunday
Upper-Body Weights	20 Minutes HIIT	Lower-Body Weights	20 Minutes HIIT	Upper-Body Weights	20 Minutes HIIT	Off

Here's an example of a schedule that may work for you. Depending on your personal schedule, figure out how to get in a few days of intensity training and strength training. It's always a good idea to take a day off to recover and give your body a break.

The Strength-Training Plan to Rebuild

+ When exercising aerobically, use the high-intensity interval-training principles. Start the exercise at a low intensity for two minutes, then increase to a moderate intensity for a minute, and finally, go to high level of intensity for 30 to 60 seconds.
+ Alternate aerobic training with strength training.
+ Train your upper body one day, then your lower body the next day you train with weights.

+ When strength training, perform five sets of an exercise, increasing the weight each set. Start with 12 repetitions, then 10–8–6 reps, then a high-intensity set.
+ Allow for one-minute rest periods between sets.

Here's a sample routine for the upper body to get you started. On Monday start with the upper body; on Wednesday train your lower body.

Upper-Body Strength Training

Do five sets each of the following exercises. As described in the "Weight Training" section of the previous chapter, each exercise consists of five sets: 12, 10, 8, 6 reps, plus a final set of 10–12 reps as your high-intensity set.

Chest	Barbell Bench Press
Back	Lat Pull-Down
Shoulders	Seated Dumbbell
Triceps	Triceps Push-Down
Biceps	Dumbbell Curl

Lower-Body Strength Training

Do five sets each of the following exercises. As described in the "Weight Training" section of the previous chapter, each exercise consists of five sets: 12, 10, 8, 6 reps, plus a final set of 10–12 reps as your high-intensity set.

Quads	Barbell Squat
Hamstrings	Lying Leg Curl
Glutes	High Knee Step-Up
Calves	Smith Machine Calf

REBUILD EXERCISE LOG
UPPER-BODY EXERCISES

EXERCISE – choose one from each group		Reps	Weight Lifted
CHEST	1. Barbell Bench Press 2. Barbell Incline Press 3. Dumbbell Bench Press	4. Incline Dumbbell Bench Press 5. Dumbbell Flye 6. Flat Bench Flye	x12	
			x10	
			x8	
	Chosen Exercise		x6	
	Intensity Set		x12	
BACK	1. Pull-Up 2. Lat Pull-Down 3. One-Arm Dumbbell Row	4. Seated Cable Row 5. Back Extension 6. Superman 7. Stability-Ball Extension	x12	
			x10	
			x8	
	Chosen Exercise		x6	
	Intensity Set		x12	
SHOULDERS	1. Seated Dumbbell Press 2. Barbell Military Press	3. Rear Dumbbell Raise 4. Barbell Upright Row 5. Dumbbell Front Raise	x12	
			x10	
			x8	
	Chosen Exercise		x6	
	Intensity Set		x12	
BICEPS	1. Standing Dumbbell Curl 2. Standing Barbell Curl	3. Preacher Curl 4. Concentration Curl 5. Cable Curl	x12	
			x10	
			x8	
	Chosen Exercise		x6	
	Intensity Set		x12	
TRICEPS	1. Seated Triceps Ext. 2. Barbell Lying Triceps Extension 3. Triceps Kickback	4. Triceps Push-Down 5. Dip 6. Dumbbell Triceps Extension	x12	
			x10	
			x8	
	Chosen Exercise		x6	
	Intensity Set		x12	

REBUILD EXERCISE LOG
LOWER-BODY EXERCISES

EXERCISE – choose one from each group		Reps	Weight Lifted
QUADRICEPS 1. Dumbbell Squat 2. Leg Press	3. Leg Extension 4. Barbell Squat	x12	
		x10	
		x8	
Chosen Exercise		x6	
Intensity Set		x12	
HAMSTRINGS 1. Lying Leg Curl 2. Lunge 3. High-Knee Step Up		x12	
		x10	
		x8	
Chosen Exercise		x6	
Intensity Set		x12	
GLUTES 1. Lunge 2. High-Knee Step Up 3. Squat		x12	
		x10	
		x8	
Chosen Exercise		x6	
Intensity Set		x12	
CALVES 1. Standing Calf Raise 2. Dumbbell Calf Raise 3. Seated Dumbbell Calf Raise		x12	
		x10	
		x8	
Chosen Exercise		x6	
Intensity Set		x12	
ABS 1. Crunch 2. Medicine-Ball Crunch	3. Stability-Ball Crunch 4. Abdominal Oblique	x12	
		x10	
		x8	
Chosen Exercise		x6	
Intensity Set		x12	

Barbell Bench Press

The barbell bench press is probably the most popular iron-pumping exercise in the gym. It is a tried-and-true exercise for building and toning your chest (pecs), the front of your shoulders, and the back of your upper arms (triceps).

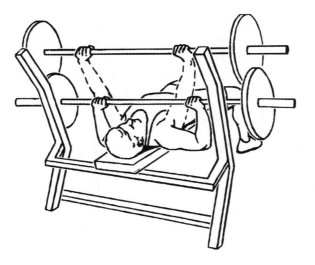

The Technique

Lie on the bench with your back flat on the bench and your feet firmly placed on the ground.

Grab the barbell above you with the grip slightly wider than your shoulders. Lift the barbell off the rack and in a slow, controlled movement, lower it to your chest about nipple height.

Just before the barbell touches your chest, press the bar upward to a locked elbow position.

Repeat the desired number of reps.

Dr. Z says ... *"Keep your feet flat on the ground and don't arch your back. Doing so may result in sprain/strain issues in the lower back."*

Dumbbell Bench Press

The dumbbell bench press is a great chest toner and builder. Besides building the muscles that fan across the chest—the pectoralis (pecs)—the press is a great exercise to strengthen other stabilizing muscles involved in daily activities.

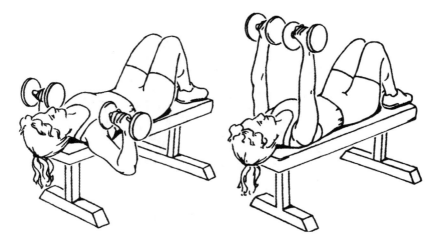

The Technique

Sit at the end of the bench with the dumbbells resting on your lower thigh. In one motion kick the weights up as you lie down on the bench. Position the dumbbells to the sides of your chest with your arms bent under each dumbbell.

Now, press the dumbbells up with the elbows until the arms are extended—where the weights now almost touch.

Lower the weights to the sides of the upper chest until you feel the pecs (chest) stretch. Repeat for the desired number of reps.

Dr. Z says . . . *"Use a full range of motion here. When you are done, don't drop the weights. Instead, twist the dumbbells so your palms are facing each other. Now while lying, lift your knees up and place weights on your knees. Push your upper body up while pressing weights into your thighs. This creates momentum to get up without dropping the weights."*

Incline Dumbbell Bench Press

Just like the flat-bench dumbbell press, the incline press is fantastic for chest development, more specifically the upper chest (pecs).

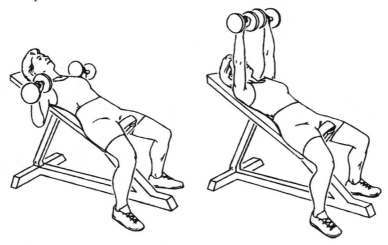

The Technique

Sit at the end of the bench with the dumbbells resting on your lower thigh. In one motion kick the weights up as you lean back on the bench. Position the dumbbells to the sides of your chest with your arms bent under each dumbbell.

Now, press the dumbbells up with your elbows until your arms are extended—where the weights now almost touch.

Lower the weights to the sides of the upper chest until you feel the chest (pecs) stretch.

Repeat for the desired number of reps.

Dr. Z says . . . *"When you're finished, don't drop the dumbbells; this foolish move may damage the rotator cuffs in your shoulders. Instead, turn the weights so your palms are facing each other; put the weights on your thighs and then stand up."*

Flat Bench Flye

Flat flyes are definitely one of my favorites for toning and building the outer, middle, and lower parts of the chest. This exercise really forces the chest muscles to work.

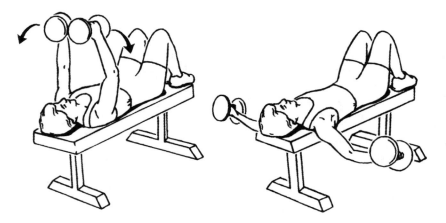

The Technique

Sit at the end of the bench with the dumbbells resting on your lower thighs. In one motion kick the weights up as you lie down on the bench. While lying on the bench, support the weights above you with your hands facing each other.

Lower the dumbbells out to your sides until the pecs are stretched, with the elbows in a slightly bent position. Once at the bottom, repeat for the desired number of reps.

> **Dr. Z says . . .** *"After your last rep, with the dumbbells now above you, bring up your knees. In one motion, drop your legs and sit up at the same time, placing the dumbbells on top of your thighs. This is a safe way to get up when you are lifting heavier weights."*

Lat Pull-Down

If you want to build a nice-looking, muscular and strong back, the lat pull-down is a key exercise. This exercise works the latissimus dorsi or "lats," which are responsible for giving the back a "V" shape. This movement also works to a lesser extent the shoulders and arms.

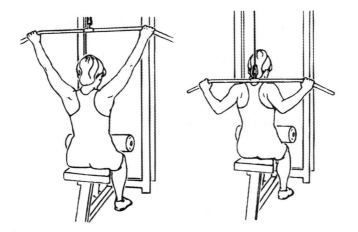

The Technique

Sit on the seat and work your knees under the thigh pads so you fit comfortably underneath them. The thigh pads prevent the weights from pulling you off the seat.

Grab the cable bar with a medium-to-wide grip. You should just about reach the bar when seated. If you can't, try adjusting the thigh pads before sitting. Grip the bar at your desired width and then let your body weight pull you down into the seat with your knees sliding under the thigh pads.

Keeping your back straight, pull the bar down to the upper part of your back. Slowly return the bar to the original position, while feeling your arms stretch up.

Dr. Z says . . . *"When pulling the weight down, try not to push your head forward. Try the same pull-down with the bar in front of your upper chest. This puts stress on the neck and joints of the shoulders."*

Pull-Up

OK, pull-ups are hard to do. But, just like the lat pull-down, the pull-up is an excellent exercise for building and strengthening your back. You can use the other back exercises to condition yourself in order to get going on the pull-up bar. Having too much weight to your body and not enough strength creates frustration when trying to do pull-ups. Get rid of the fat and build and strengthen your body so you can add this to your routine.

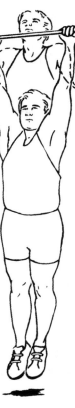

The Technique

This is pretty straightforward.

Grab the pull-up bar with your hands placed about shoulder-width apart and your palms facing away from you.

Pull yourself upward until your chin is over the bar. Complete the exercise by slowly moving to the hanging position, so your arms and shoulders are fully extended.

Repeat for the desired number of reps.

Dr. Z says . . . "*Accomplishing a pull-up is empowering. Strive to do not only one, but sets of them that are part of your routine. Gyms have pull-up assisted machines to help you get strong enough to do them on your own. As Nike says . . . just do it!*"

Seated Cable Row

The seated cable row is another one of those "must do" exercises for training the muscles of the back. Like the squat for your legs, the cable row is a great compound exercise. Compound exercises are multi-joint movements that involve action and stability from many muscle groups. The cable row hits the lats, postural muscles, rear shoulder muscles overlying the shoulder blades, and muscles in the arms.

The Technique

Sit on the bench with your hips back and your knees slightly bent, with your feet vertical on the platform. Now reach for the handles of the bar or cable attachment. You will feel a slight stretch in your hamstrings and low back.

Pull the cable attachment to your lower chest and at the same time straighten yourself up— all in one movement. While pulling, pull your shoulders back and push your chest forward while slightly arching your back.

Then, return the cable attachment back to the starting position so your arms are extended, your shoulders are stretched, and your low back is flexed forward.

Repeat for desired number of reps.

Dr. Z says ... *"Try not to hyperextend when pulling back or round your back when extending your arms. This can put unnecessary force into the joints of your spine and aggravate any back problems you may have."*

Superman

The Man of Steel is not the only one who can have great posture. This is a great exercise to strengthen the muscles of the lower back, as well as to tone your glutes and hamstrings. Don't be fooled; this exercise is harder than it looks, but it is a must-do exercise.

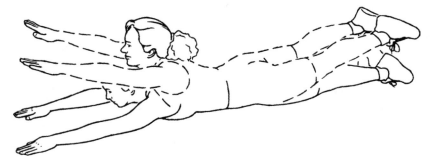

The Technique

Lie face down on the floor with your arms extended and your legs together—also extended. Keep your head and neck in a neutral position.

Keeping your limbs straight and your upper body stationary; simultaneously lift your arms and legs up toward the ceiling, forming a curve with your body. Exhale as you lift your legs and arms. Hold for a count of 10 and don't forget to breathe. Inhale and lower your limbs to the ground to complete a rep.

Repeat for the desired number of reps.

Dr. Z says . . . *"This is a great exercise for anyone suffering from back problems. It helps to restore normal joint movement and strengthens the muscles that support the spine, making it a great therapeutic exercise."*

Stability-Ball Extension

An alternative to the Superman exercises is extension on a stability ball. This exercise not only provides some stability because you're leaning over a yoga ball, it is also hitting the back of your shoulder (or rear delts) and the muscles of the middle back. This is another great posture builder.

The Technique

Kneel on the ground and lean over an exercise ball while grabbing dumbbells placed next to the ball. Raise your torso away from the ball; at the same time, lift your arms up and away from the ball.

Return your torso (upper body) to the ball and repeat for the desired number of reps.

> **Dr. Z says . . .** *"When lifting your arms, rotate your hands so your palms are facing down holding the weights in a horizontal position. The obvious hazard here is letting the ball roll away from you during the exercise. Pay attention. To prevent the ball from rolling away from you, wedge a pair of shoes under the front edge."*

Back Extension

Just like the Superman exercise, back extension on a bench is a great way to strengthen your lower back and postural muscles.

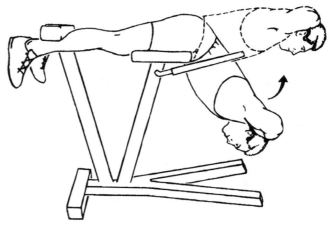

The Technique

Before getting on the bench, set the height of the pads no higher than the top of your pelvis (bones of your waist).

Get yourself into position on the back-extension bench by standing in front of the pads, then resting your thighs on the pads while securing your feet behind you. Ask for assistance if you are unsure.

Start with your back and spine straight. Slowly lower your upper body down until your upper body is pointing to the ground. Now raise yourself back up to the starting position using the low-back muscles in a slow, controlled movement.

Dr. Z says . . . *"Don't force yourself up too far, forcing an exaggerated curve in your low back. To do so may stress the joints in your low back, causing a sprain/strain issue and pain."*

Barbell Military Press

One of the best exercises for shoulder development and strength is the military press. For many years, the press was a measure of your upper-body power, and it still is today. When effectively executed, the military press works mainly the shoulders, and secondly the triceps (back of the arm) and your abs.

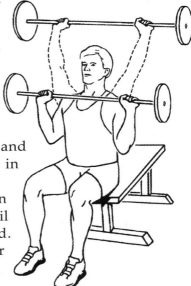

The Technique

Grab a barbell with an overhand grip slightly wider than your shoulders and sit on a bench. Position the barbell in front of your upper chest.

With your feet firmly planted on the ground, press the bar upward until your arms are extended overhead. Exhale as you lift. Lower the bar back to the chest. To give yourself a little more strength through the lift, tighten up your abs.

Repeat for the desired number of reps.

> **Dr. Z says . . .** *"You can perform this standing, or seated in front of a Smith machine. If you have low-back problems, you are better off doing this one seated."*

Dumbbell Front Raise

Along with looking good, the front of the shoulders or "front delts" are involved with activities of daily living like lifting a grocery bag or briefcase. The key to this exercise is form, so use light weights and slow, controlled movement.

The Technique

Grasp dumbbells in both hands and position them in front of the upper legs with your elbows straight or slightly bent.

Raise the dumbbells forward and upward until your arms are above horizontal. Exhale as you lift. Then, slowly lower the weight back down to the starting position.

Repeat for the desired number of reps.

Dr. Z says . . . *"Focus on moving only your shoulders, and avoid swinging the weights. That can injure your shoulders and low back."*

Rear Dumbbell Raise

Not all shoulder exercises are created equal. Most people train the front and the side deltoids, neglecting the rear deltoid. There are three heads to the deltoid muscle— front, medial, and posterior. All three need to be trained equally if you want nice, well-rounded shoulders.

The Technique

Grab dumbbells and sit at the end of a bench with your feet placed beyond your knees. While bent over with your torso on your thighs, position the dumbbells behind your feet. Grip the dumbbells with a slight bend in your elbows and your palms facing down.

Begin by raising your arms to the sides until your elbows are at shoulder height. Maintain the fixed position of your elbows, and maintain the upper arm perpendicular throughout the movement.

Lower and repeat for the desired number of reps.

> **Dr. Z says . . .** *"Keep your torso against your thighs. If you position your torso at, say, 45 degrees, you are not targeting the rear deltoid. Keep your body down and your feet forward, forcing your torso down on your thighs."*

Barbell Upright Row

The upright row is one of the best compound exercises emphasizing the upper traps (the "massage-my-shoulders" muscles) and the deltoids. The upright row can help you fully develop the shoulders and trapezius muscles evenly.

The Technique

With an overhand grip, pick up a barbell with your hands shoulder-width apart.

Keep your back straight and eyes facing forward. Now, lift the barbell straight up with your elbows leading. Allow your wrists to flex as the bar rises.

Lower and repeat for the desired number of reps.

Dr. Z says . . . *"Focus on keeping your elbows higher than your forearms. Also, don't lean forward or back, because the movement of your body makes the exercise easier. At the top, pause and squeeze the traps and shoulders for a little more intensity."*

Barbell Curl

The barbell curl is the meat-and-potatoes exercise for your biceps, and it is a favorite exercise because of the high visibility your upper arms get. As it sounds, the biceps comprise two heads—the short head and the long head.

The Technique

While standing upright, grip a barbell with palms up, just beyond shoulder width, and elbows to your sides.

While holding your upper arm stationary, curl the bar up until it is at shoulder level. Exhale as you lift.

When the bar is being lifted, you should feel the front of your upper arm or biceps contract.

Once completed, slowly lower the bar to the starting position for the next repetition.

Repeat for desired number of reps.

Dr. Z says . . . *"Form is key here! To help lift the weight, many people sway during the lift, which can injure your lower back. To prevent this, tighten up your abs during both lifting up and lowering down of the bar."*

Concentration Curl

The concentration curl is a fantastic exercise for isolating just the biceps. It is the exercise of choice for maximum biceps stimulation, as well as to build the peak of the biceps. Because you can isolate the biceps, you can use it to resolve any asymmetries in your arms, for example, if one arm is bigger than the other.

The Technique

Sit on a bench with feet apart. Grasp a dumbbell between your feet while placing the back of your left upper arm to your left inside thigh.

Raise (curl) the dumbbell to the front shoulder. Then lower the dumbbell until the arm is fully extended.

Repeat for the desired number of reps, then switch arms.

Dr. Z says ... *"Breathe out when curling the weight. At the top of the contraction, hold the position for a second as you squeeze the biceps. Avoid swinging motions at any time."*

Preacher Curl

The preacher curl is a variation of the barbell curl that you do sitting on a curl bench. This is also a great exercise to isolate the biceps for strength and building the upper arm. As a variation, this can also be done with single dumbbells.

The Technique

Set up your barbell on the preacher bench. Sit on the bench and grab the bar, palms up and shoulder-width apart.

Raise (curl) the bar until the forearms are vertical; at the same time, squeeze the biceps. Now, slowly lower the barbell until your arms are fully extended.

Repeat for the desired number of reps.

Dr. Z says . . . *"When lowering the barbell, be careful not to overextend your elbows. This can cause stress on the lower biceps tendon where it attaches near the elbow. Right at the bottom of the movement, leave a slight bend in your arms to take away the physical stress put on the tendons."*

Triceps Push-Down

The triceps push-down is one of the best exercises to build the back of the arm (triceps). Like it sounds, the triceps comprises the three different heads that give the classic "horseshoe" appearance when the arm is extended. This is a great exercise to help the "turkey-arm" syndrome.

The Technique

While facing the triceps machine, grasp the cable bar with an overhand grip. The starting point is about chest level.

Keep your feet at or slightly wider than shoulder width, and keep your elbows to your sides.

Start with light weights to see how this exercise works.

Brace your body by tightening up your stomach (abs). Now push down on the handle until your elbows are fully extended.

Allow the bar to come back to a starting point with a controlled movement.

Repeat for desired number of reps.

Dr. Z says . . . *"Bend your knees slightly while you push down on the bar, and stay upright as much as possible. Try not to bend forward too much while pushing down, as this might be rough on your shoulders and lower back."*

Barbell Lying Triceps Extension

The lying triceps extension is one of the best triceps builders there is. Period. During this exercise, most people have a tendency to let their elbows flare out. Before you start, remember to keep your elbows in, and don't lock your elbows at the top of the movement. By doing so, you take tension away from the triceps, the muscles you are trying to build.

The Technique

Lie on your back on a bench so your head is at the end of the bench. With a barbell on the ground at the head of the bench, reach back and grasp the barbell with palms facing up. Lift the barbell up so it's positioned over your forehead with your arms extended.

With the arms fully extended, lower the bar by bending the elbows. As the bar comes close to your head, bring it back slightly so it just clears the curvature of your head. Now, as the bar clears your head, extend the arms fully. Repeat for the desired number of reps.

Dr. Z says . . . *"Inhale as you lower the bar by bending at the elbows, and exhale as you push the bar up to an extended-arm position. Only your forearms should move; your upper arms should remain stationary."*

Dumbbell Triceps Extension

Here's another triceps isolation exercise. Among all the triceps exercises to choose from, this particular movement is sure to tone and build the back of your arms. The key to getting the benefits out of this exercise is form.

The Technique

Sit on a seat or bench. While holding a dumbbell in your left hand, position the dumbbell overhead with your arm straight up or slightly back. At the same time, take your opposite hand and support the back of the arm to be extended. This helps prevent movement of the whole arm when extending.

Lower the dumbbell behind the neck or shoulder while maintaining your upper arm's vertical position throughout the exercise. Extend the arm until your arm is straight.

Repeat for the desired number of reps, and then switch arms.

Dr. Z says . . . "When you lower the dumbbell, let it pull your arm down and back to get a nice stretch in the triceps. If done correctly, you should feel this only in the triceps."

Dip

The dip is a great compound movement that works multiple muscles in the upper body, like the chest, shoulder, and triceps. You can use the dip to build your chest muscles, or you can use it as a triceps exercise.

The Technique

Get up on the parallel bars with your torso perpendicular to the floor. This will isolate the triceps. If you lean forward, you will emphasize your chest and shoulders.

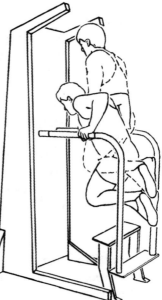

While supporting yourself, bend your knees and cross your feet behind you. Slowly lower your body until your shoulder joints are just even with your elbows. Now, push back up until your elbows are nearly straight but not locked.

Repeat for the desired number of reps.

Dr. Z says . . . *"For some, this may be tough on the shoulders and pecs. If you are feeling pain with this movement, consider another exercise. If you have no pain or pre-existing shoulder problem, the dip is superb for the triceps, chest, and shoulders."*

Barbell Squat

If you're not squatting, you're not training. The squat is a superb exercise that targets not only the upper thighs (quads) and the buttocks or glutes; it works the whole body. The major bonus with this exercise is that it not only burns a lot of calories; it burns fat. Squats can be done with a barbell as seen, on a Smith machine, and holding dumbbells or kettle bells.

The Technique

Place the barbell just above your shoulders, resting it on the upper-back or trapezius muscles. If that is uncomfortable, wrap towel around the bar to protect your upper back.

Stand with your feet roughly shoulder-width apart and slightly turned out.

Bend your knees and lower into a squat position. Stop when your knees are at 90 degrees. Try to keep the natural curve in the low back.

Stabilize the bar with your upper body, and push with your legs and glutes to a standing position while keeping your knees in line with your toes.

Repeat for desired number of reps.

Dr. Z says . . . *"Always start light; you can add weight as you learn good form and get stronger. Make sure your knees line up with your feet, which are slightly pointed out. When coming down, try to maintain the curve in your low back. If the weight is too heavy, it will force your back into an unnatural position."*

Leg Press

The leg press is a compound movement to strengthen your quads (thighs) and glutes (butt). This is a great exercise to prepare you for all sports, including skiing, biking, sprinting, and all other activities that require lower-body strength.

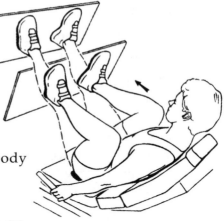

The Technique

After putting weighted plates on the machine, sit with your back on padded support. Place your feet on the platform. The higher you place your feet, the more hamstring and glute involvement; the lower your foot placement, the more quad involvement. Push with your feet, extending your hips and knees. Release the dock (support) lever and grab the handle to the sides.

Lower the sled by flexing your hips and knees until your knees are close to your chest. At the bottom of this movement, push to extend your knees and hips.

Repeat for the desired number or reps.

Dr. Z says . . . *"To prevent excessive stress on your knees and low back, avoid lowering your legs too close to your torso. Allow your thighs to touch the outside of your lower ribs."*

Leg Extension

If you are looking to build and shape the front of your thighs, leg extensions will get the job done.

The Technique

Sit on the machine with your back against the padded support. Place the front of your lower legs under the padded lever. The back of your knees should be positioned at the front end of the seat. Grasp the side handles for support and to keep yourself on the seat.

Extend your legs until your knees are straight. Hold that for a count of three, and then slowly return the padded lever to its original position by bending your knees.

> **Dr. Z says . . .** "To avoid issues with your knees or low back, make sure your back is firmly pressed against the seat back. While lifting, don't wobble or sway side to side. Adjust the lower limb pads so they are not too far up your shins. Don't do this exercise if your knees hurt."

Lying Leg Curl

Having great thighs doesn't mean a thing if you don't have nice hamstrings. The lying leg curl is an isolated exercise used to tone and build the backs of your thighs. The hamstrings are the legs' biceps.

The Technique

Position your body on the leg-curl machine facing down. Adjust the leg pads, so they are at the lowest part of your calves.

Grab the handles on the bench, and pull the weight up toward your body. Feel the hamstring contract, and squeeze at the top position.

From the top position, slowly lower the weight back down to the starting position.

Repeat for desired number of reps.

Dr. Z says . . . *"Use the full range of motion here, by curling the weight as high as possible—almost until the pads are touching your buttocks. Allow yourself the full stretch at the bottom."*

Standing Calf Raise

Calves—either you got 'em or you don't. Those who didn't inherit the calf gene are going to need to do a little work. The calf muscles—gastrocnemius and soleus—are tough to develop and, therefore, require very specific training. The standing calf raise is the gold standard in calf development.

The Technique

Standing calf raises can be done on a Smith machine (as shown), on a standing calf machine, off a step, or by holding dumbbells. When executing Smith machine heel raises, set the bar on the Smith machine to shoulder height. Put a step or calf block below the bar.

Step on the block and position the balls of your feet on the edge, pointing your toes slightly inward. Get yourself under the Smith bar, so the bar is across your shoulders. Now, push the weight off the rack, and drop your heels down as far as possible. Slowly raise your heels as high as you can go, squeezing your calf muscles at the top. Slowly lower your heels back to the starting position.

Repeat for the desired number of reps.

Dr. Z says . . . *"When lowering your heels, don't bounce or come down too hard, as this may put too much stress on the Achilles tendon. Squeeze your calves at the top for maximum effect."*

Seated Dumbbell Calf Raise

The calves contain deep muscle (soleus) and superficial muscle (gastrocnemius) that you see when the calves contract. The soleus gives the calf width, while the gastrocs give the calf the diamond shape. The seated dumbbell calf raise is the best way to add some girth to your calves.

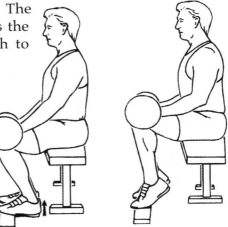

The Technique

Sit on the edge of a bench and place the balls of your feet on a 2x4 or a step platform. Place a pair of dumbbells on top of both knees. Lower your heels as low as you can to feel the stretch. Push off with your toes, lifting your heels while contracting the calves.

Lower heels to the starting position again. Repeat for the desired number of reps. If you need heavier weights, find the seated calf bench.

Dr. Z says . . . "*The calves are dense and super-strong, so make sure you stress them. When dropping your heels, go slow and don't bounce. To do so may injure your Achilles tendon.*"

Medicine-Ball Crunch

Here's another variation of the crunch for your abdominals. This is a little more challenging because you are holding a weighted medicine ball. Try this with a four-, six-, or eight-pound ball.

The Technique

Hold a small medicine ball against your chest. Position yourself with feet flat on the ground and knees slightly shoulder-width apart.

Contract your abs while holding the ball against your chest; at the same time, exhale. As you exhale, really squeeze your abs; hold for a second or two, then slowly lower yourself back down.

Repeat for the desired number of reps.

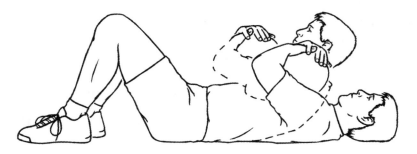

Dr. Z says . . . *"Again, form is key here. When raising your chest, contract those abs while exhaling. You are sure to get a good 'burn.'"*

Stability-Ball Crunch

For those with low-back issues, this is a great alternative to floor crunches.

The Technique

Sit back on an exercise ball while securing it to the floor. Keep your feet and knees shoulder-width apart, and interlock your fingers behind your head.

While holding yourself in place on the ball, contract your abs, raising yourself about 30 degrees. Exhale on the way up, and inhale on the way back.

> **Dr. Z says . . .** *"When performing the crunch, keep from moving on the ball. Just use it to support yourself. Exhale when you crunch, and inhale on the way back."*

Abdominal Oblique

To tone and develop sexy abs, you need to work the muscles on the sides of the abdominals (the obliques). If you have "love handles," that fat has covered this important muscle group. If you are a woman looking for the hourglass figure, or a gent who wants that "V" shape, get to work on your obliques.

The Technique

Sit on an exercise ball. Walk forward with your feet to position the ball in the middle of your back. At the same time, interlock your fingers and place your hands behind your head. Your head should be positioned horizontally to your body.

In this position, contract your abdominals and flex at the waist. At the same time, twist slightly, bringing your left elbow toward the opposite side of your body.

Repeat for the desired number of reps, changing sides. The crunches can also be done alternating: left to right, right to left.

Dr. Z says . . . *"Don't pull on your head or neck; use your abs. To really work your abs and obliques, try holding a weight or medicine ball (5–10 pounds) against your chest. Holding the weight, contract your abs while exhaling."*

RECIPES

Before you get started with the delicious recipes, the following chart will show how flexible they can be. Some recipes work well early in the day, while some are best suited for lunch or dinner.

You can mix and match to create more variety. That way you know, no matter what time of day, what you're eating is just right!

KEY: B = Breakfast; L = Lunch; D = Dinner; S = Snack

	B	L	D	S
Ambrosia Fruit Salad	√			√
Asian Red Slaw	√	√	√	√
Bison Burgers with Salsa	√	√	√	
Blueberry Smoothie	√			√
Broccoli Rabe		√	√	
Chester's Chili		√	√	
Chicken Sausage / Sweet Potato One-Pot Wonder		√	√	
Chinese Chicken		√	√	
Chunky Vegetable Soup		√	√	
Crispy Cruciferous Salad	√	√	√	√
Curried Chicken Salad	√	√	√	
Devilicious Curried Eggs (with variations)	√			√
Dr. Z's Fast & Easy Snacks				√
Dr. Z's "Just Wing It" Salads		√	√	
Dr. Z's Zesty Stir-Fry		√	√	
Egg & Avocado on Toast	√			
Egg & Olive Salad	√	√		√
Eggplant Tapenade				√
Fantastic Spinach	√	√	√	
Feisty Breakfast Medley	√			
Fresh Fruit & Mint Salad	√	√		√
Grilled Kabobs—Chicken, Beef, or Lamb		√	√	
Guacamole	√	√	√	√

	B	L	D	S
Hearty Navy-Bean Soup		√	√	√
Hummus				√
Jalapeño-Apple Salsa				√
Kale & White-Bean Soup		√	√	√
Kitchen Sink Soup		√	√	√
Lemon-Fresh Quinoa with Herbs	√	√	√	√
Magic Color-Changing Shrimp Stir-Fry		√	√	
Mango & Black-Bean Salsa	√	√	√	√
Manhattan Clam Chowder		√	√	
Marinated Chicken Kabobs		√	√	
Middle-Eastern Burger		√	√	
Mushroom & Broccoli Frittata	√	√	√	
Poached Fish Pouches		√	√	
Power Oatmeal (with variations)	√			
Power Pasta		√		
Quick Lemon Chicken		√	√	
Quinoa Tabouleh	√	√	√	√
Red Cabbage, Onions, & Oranges		√	√	
Roasted Brussels Sprouts		√	√	√
Salmon Salad		√		√
Sautéed Salmon & Green Beans		√	√	
Scrambled Eggs & Sundried Tomatoes	√			
Seafood Lettuce Tacos		√	√	
Sesame Broccoli		√	√	
Spaghetti Carbonara		√		
Spanish Stuffed Peppers		√	√	
Spiced Sweet-Potato Cubes	√	√	√	
Spicy Garlic Hummus				√
Split-Pea Soup		√	√	
Stewed Beef Shank (or Lamb Shank)		√	√	

	B	L	D	S
String Beans & Tomatoes		√	√	
Summer Fruit Salad	√	√	√	√
Summer Poached Salmon		√	√	
Summer Salad		√	√	
Super-Moist Turkey Meatballs		√	√	√
Sweet Mushroom Salad		√	√	√
Taco-Less Taco Salad		√	√	
Tangy Salsa & Eggs	√			
Thai Curried Tilapia (or Chicken)		√	√	
Tomato Relish				√
Tomato Soup		√	√	√
Tuna Salad		√	√	√
Turkey & Vegetable One-Dish Supper		√	√	
Turkey Bolognese			√	
Turkey (or Beef) Confetti Bowl		√	√	
Tuscan Bean Dip				√
Tuscan Cabbage, Kale, & Beans	√	√	√	
Vegetable Stir-Fry			√	√
Waldorf Salad	√	√		
Zucchini Pancakes	√	√		

RECIPES TO BE USED ONLY AS A TREAT:

Flourless Almond-Butter Cookies				√
Gluten-Free Banana Muffins				√

A list of product recommendations and resources, including website links, is located after the recipe section. Use that if you are looking for grass-fed meat or wild seafood, or any of the brand-name products I've recommended.

AMBROSIA FRUIT SALAD

SERVES 4

CALORIES PER SERVING: 188

INGREDIENTS
2 tablespoons shredded unsweetened coconut
¼ cup orange juice
1 large orange
1 small banana, sliced lengthwise, then crosswise
1 cup sliced green grapes
½ cup chopped raw pecans

DIRECTIONS
Combine orange juice and shredded coconut; set aside until the coconut softens (about ½ hour). Remove segments from the orange and break them into bite-sized chunks. In a bowl, combine the fruit and pecans. Drain the shredded coconut and mix into the fruit salad.

ASIAN RED SLAW

This is an excellent accompaniment to any grilled food. The anti-oxidants in red cabbage will help to offset free-radical damage from eating charred food.

SERVES 6

CALORIES PER SERVING: 187

INGREDIENTS

1 small head red cabbage, shredded
½ head Savoy cabbage, shredded
1 can water chestnuts, drained and sliced
1–2 large carrots, shredded
2 green onions, thinly sliced
3 tablespoons toasted sesame seeds
¼ cup slivered almonds

Dressing
1 tablespoon sesame oil
1 tablespoon extra-virgin olive oil (cold-pressed)
1 tablespoon organic tamari soy sauce
¼ cup rice-wine vinegar
1 tablespoon agave syrup

DIRECTIONS

In a jar, combine all dressing ingredients. Shake vigorously to mix well; set aside.

In a large bowl, combine all vegetables until evenly distributed. To preserve the crunchy texture, add dressing just before serving. Garnish with toasted sesame seeds and slivered almonds.

BEEF SHANK (or Lamb Shank)

SERVES 4

CALORIES PER SERVING: 253

INGREDIENTS
¾ cup freshly squeezed orange juice
1 tablespoon garlic powder
1 tablespoon onion powder
1 teaspoon pink Himalayan salt
1 teaspoon freshly ground black pepper
2–4 large beef (or lamb) shanks
1 15-ounce can organic stewed tomatoes, sliced
½ cup red wine
1 teaspoon thyme
2 bay leaves
1 medium yellow onion, sliced
4 stalks celery, sliced
3 carrots, sliced
10 large cremini mushrooms, sliced

DIRECTIONS
In a large bowl, combine orange juice, garlic powder, onion powder, salt, and pepper. Add the meat; stir to be sure all the meat is covered. Marinate for a couple of hours.

Preheat oven to 350°. Arrange the shanks in a Dutch oven. Add the marinade and tomatoes (with juice), wine, thyme, and bay leaves. Cover and bake for 1½ hours. Remove from oven; add sliced onion, celery, carrots, and mushrooms. Add salt and pepper to taste; return to oven for another 1½ hours.

Serve over brown rice or quinoa for a more substantial meal.

BISON BURGERS WITH SALSA

SERVES 4

CALORIES PER SERVING: 337

INGREDIENTS
1 pound ground bison
⅓ cup unsweetened mild salsa
(Green Mountain is a good brand)

DIRECTIONS
In a mixing bowl, combine bison and salsa; mix thoroughly. The best way to do this is to mix it with your hands. Form the mixture into burgers; there should enough to make four 4-ounce burgers. Grill to your preference.

VARIATION
This same recipe makes a great meatloaf.

Preheat oven to 350°. In a large bowl, combine two pounds ground meat—bison, beef, turkey, or any other grass-fed meat—with ½ to ¾ cup salsa. Bake for 40 minutes to an hour, or until the internal temperature is 160°.

BLUEBERRY SMOOTHIE

This is an excellent pre- or post-workout snack.
SERVES 1
CALORIES PER SERVING: 157

INGREDIENTS
½ small banana
1 cup blueberries
1 scoop powdered greens*
1 scoop protein powder (whey, egg-white, or rice protein)
1 cup water

DIRECTIONS
Put all ingredients in a blender (or Vitamix®) and blend until desired consistency. If it's too thick, use a little more water. If it's too watery, use less water.

This is perfect for after a workout. Depending on the grams of protein per scoop, you may have to add more protein powder. I use a micro-filtered whey protein called Unipro's Perfect Protein** made by a division of Metagenics. One scoop has 16 grams of protein. I usually use 1½ scoops after my workout.

*nutraMetrix® Complete Greens can be ordered from my website.
**Metagenics® Perfect Protein can be ordered from my website.

BROCCOLI RABE

SERVES 2–3

CALORIES PER SERVING: 139 FOR 2; 93 FOR 3

INGREDIENTS
1 bunch broccoli rabe
1 tablespoon olive oil
2 shallots or 1 small onion, finely diced
½ bulb garlic, smashed and roughly chopped
¼ cup raisins (optional)
~ Salt and pepper to taste
~ Pinch of red-pepper flakes (optional)

DIRECTIONS
Wash broccoli rabe very well, leaving some water in the leaves. Cut away lower half of stems, and cut the bunch into 3 sections. In a large skillet over medium heat, add broccoli rabe with 8 ounces water and sprinkle with salt. Steam until just tender and still bright green; do not overcook. Transfer broccoli rabe to a bowl and set aside. In the same skillet, add oil, shallots (or onion), and garlic; cook until light golden. Do not burn; add a bit more oil if needed. Add broccoli rabe and liquid; cook for 2 minutes. Add salt and pepper to taste and red-pepper flakes, if desired.

CHESTER'S CHILI

Chili is a perfect meal to warm you up on cool autumn nights. You can substitute ground turkey or bison for the grass-fed beef.
SERVES 6

CALORIES PER SERVING: 216

INGREDIENTS
1 tablespoon grapeseed oil
2 medium onions, chopped
1 cup chopped green bell pepper
1 pound grass-fed ground beef
1 28-ounce can diced tomatoes
1 8-ounce can tomato sauce
2 teaspoons chili powder
1 teaspoon sea salt
½ teaspoon paprika
⅛ teaspoon cayenne pepper
1 15-ounce can red kidney beans, drained

DIRECTIONS
In a soup pot over medium heat, sauté chopped onions in grapeseed oil until soft. Add the chopped green pepper and cook another couple of minutes. Add the ground beef; stir together with onions and green pepper until the meat is cooked through. Stir in the remaining ingredients, except for the kidney beans.

Turn the heat down and simmer for an hour, stirring occasionally. Skim off extra liquid with a soup ladle. After about one hour, turn off heat and add the kidney beans. Mix well and serve.

CHICKEN SAUSAGE & SWEET POTATO ONE-POT WONDER

SERVES 6

CALORIES PER SERVING: 374

INGREDIENTS

3 large sweet potatoes
1 bulb fennel, sliced (optional)
6 links chicken sausage, sliced ¼-inch thick
1 large Vidalia onion, cut in quarters and ¼-inch slices
1–1½ cups frozen green peas, thawed
3 tablespoons grapeseed oil
2 teaspoons sea salt
2 teaspoons fennel powder (substitute dried oregano if
    preferred)

DIRECTIONS

Cook sweet potatoes 8–15 minutes in a microwave. Cut in half; set aside to cool enough to handle. Cut into ½-inch slices, keeping the skin intact. Salt and pepper to taste and set aside to cool completely.

Steam sliced fennel until tender but firm. Drain and cut into bite-sized pieces. Omit this if you do not like the flavor of fennel.

In a large skillet over medium heat, add 1 tablespoon grapeseed oil and sliced onion; sauté for 3 minutes, stirring frequently. Add salt and pepper to taste, fennel powder (or dried oregano), and peas; sauté for another 5 minutes. When the peas and onions are a bit browned, remove from the set aside.

Using the same pan, add 2 tablespoons grapeseed oil and sliced sausages; cook until browned (most chicken sausages are precooked). Add onions and peas, steamed fennel (if desired), and sweet potatoes. Toss gently for 3–4 minutes until flavors combine.

CHICKEN STIR-FRY (or shrimp)

SERVES 6 • CALORIES PER SERVING: 240

INGREDIENTS
2–3 tablespoons grapeseed oil
1 pound organic chicken cut into strips
    (or shrimp, if you prefer)
~ Bragg Liquid Aminos (see Resources)
    (or organic tamari soy sauce)
1 medium white onion, chopped
1½ cups chopped asparagus
1½ cups chopped broccoli
1 cup chopped carrots, cut in slivers
1 cup chopped zucchini
1 cup chopped mushrooms (white, maitake, or shiitake)
¾ cup chopped snow peas
½–¾ cup chopped bell peppers (red, green, yellow, orange)
1 tablespoon minced ginger root
1 tablespoon minced garlic
1 teaspoon sesame seed oil (optional)

DIRECTIONS
In a 13-inch stainless-steel wok over medium to high heat, add 1 tablespoon grapeseed oil. When the oil is hot, add chicken strips and small amount of Bragg Liquid Aminos (or organic tamari soy sauce). Stir constantly while cooking until the chicken is coated with the sauce and slightly pink on the inside. Remove chicken from the wok and set aside.

Add 1–2 tablespoons grapeseed oil and onion to the wok; sauté until onion is soft. Add asparagus, broccoli, and carrots, along with a splash of Bragg Liquid Aminos. Once the vegetables are soft, add the remaining vegetables. Stir-fry until the vegetables are the consistency you like.

Add ginger and garlic; stir-fry 1 or 2 more minutes. If more liquid is needed, add more amino acids. Add the chicken; stir-fry until warmed. At the last minute, stir in 1 teaspoon sesame-seed oil for flavor.

Make brown rice ahead of time. Serve the stir-fry over ½ cup of brown rice for a substantial meal.

CHINESE CHICKEN

SERVES 4

CALORIES PER SERVING: 390 WITHOUT RICE; 404 WITH RICE

INGREDIENTS
1 whole plump chicken (3–4 pounds)*
2 carrots
1 onion
4 celery stalks

Ginger Sauce
¼ cup chopped ginger
1 bunch scallions, chopped (light and dark green only)
½ cup grapeseed oil
~ Sea salt to taste

Rice
1½ cups uncooked brown Jasmine rice
4 tablespoons oyster sauce (thin with water if desired)

DIRECTIONS
In a large pot, completely submerse the chicken in water; add sea salt to taste and cover. Bring the water to a boil, turn off heat, and let stand covered for 20 minutes. Repeat that step two more times. Pull one chicken leg back; if it moves easily and the liquid in the joint runs clear, the chicken is done. Remove from the pot and set it aside to rest. When it's cooled enough to touch, pull it apart into bite-sized pieces.

Cook rice according to package directions.

In a food processor, puree ginger to a fine gritty texture. Add chopped scallions and grapeseed oil; process until smooth. Add salt to taste.

To serve, pay attention to the amount of each ingredient. Start with ¾ cup rice. Add a bit of oyster sauce; use sparingly, as it is very strong. Add 3–4 ounces chicken (the size of the palm of your hand) and top with a little ginger sauce. Use the sauce sparingly, as it is high in calories.

Use the chicken stock from this recipe to make the Kitchen Sink Soup, or any other dish calling for chicken stock. Use the leftover chicken in the soup or to make chicken salad.

CHUNKY VEGETABLE SOUP

This is a very versatile recipe. Use the recommended ingredients or whatever you have. Frozen vegetables work well in this recipe.
SERVES 4–6

CALORIES PER SERVING: 182 FOR 4; 121 FOR 6

INGREDIENTS
2–3 tablespoons grapeseed oil
1 onion, diced
2 carrots, sliced
2 celery stalks, sliced
4 cups water
4 cups organic, low-sodium vegetable broth
15-ounce can diced tomatoes
2 garlic cloves, minced (1 tablespoon of minced
    garlic from a jar)
1 cup green beans, cut into bite-sized pieces
1 small sweet potato, diced
½ cup fresh or frozen peas
1 cup chopped cabbage, kale, or collard greens
1 tablespoon dried herbs (thyme, rosemary, tarragon)
1 tablespoon miso (optional)
½ cup fresh parsley, minced
~ Sea salt and black pepper to taste

DIRECTIONS
In a large soup pot, add grapeseed oil, onions, carrots, and celery; sauté until onions are soft. Add water, vegetable broth, tomatoes, garlic, green beans, sweet potato, and the rest of the ingredients. Simmer until all vegetables are soft. Season with sea salt and black pepper.

CRISPY CRUCIFEROUS SALAD

SERVES 6

CALORIES PER SERVING: 250

INGREDIENTS

Salad
1 large head (2 pounds) broccoli
¾ head cauliflower
2 large carrots, shredded
¼ head red cabbage, finely chopped
5 radishes, sliced
1 cup snap peas or snow peas, sliced
½ small red onion, sliced (or 2 scallions, thinly sliced)
½ bunch flat-leaf parsley, chopped
½ cup pumpkin seeds or slivered raw almonds

Dressing
¼ cup extra virgin olive oil
4 tablespoons rice vinegar (or apple-cider vinegar)
2 teaspoons agave syrup
~ Freshly ground black pepper
1–2 teaspoons sea salt
1 sprig fresh lemon thyme, chopped

DIRECTIONS

Cut broccoli and cauliflower into bite-sized pieces. In a large bowl, mix all salad ingredients together. In a second bowl, whisk together all dressing ingredients. Add the dressing to the salad; mix well. Add salt to taste. Chill before serving. Stir often to create more liquid; this will have the effect of marinating the vegetables.

CURRIED CHICKEN SALAD

SERVES 6–8

CALORIES PER SERVING: 367 FOR 6; 275 FOR 8

INGREDIENTS

4 large chicken breasts, boneless and skinless
½–¾ cup mayonnaise (or Vegenaise®—see Resources)
2 teaspoons dehydrated onion, finely chopped (or ½ small
    red onion)
2 tablespoons curry powder
4 stalks celery, sliced lengthwise and cut into ¼-inch pieces
½–¾ cup raisins (or dried cranberries)
~ Sea salt
~ Freshly ground black pepper

DIRECTIONS

Steam chicken breasts until done. After cooling, cut into bite-
sized pieces. Set aside in a large bowl.

In a small bowl, combine mayonnaise, chopped onion, and
curry powder. Add to the chicken and mix well. (The amount
of mayonnaise will depend on the amount of chicken.) Add
celery, raisins, salt, and pepper, and mix well. Serve over a bed
of endive or radicchio lettuce.

VARIATION

Roasted turkey breast can be substituted for chicken. Cut
an equivalent amount of turkey into bite-sized pieces, and
continue with directions in the second paragraph above.

DEVILICIOUS CURRIED EGGS

SERVING = 2 EGGS (4 HALVES) AS BREAKFAST;
1 EGG (2 HALVES) AS A SNACK
CALORIES PER SERVING: 267 BREAKFAST; 133 SNACK

INGREDIENTS
12 eggs, hard-boiled
¾ cup mayonnaise (or Vegenaise®—see Resources)
1 tablespoon spicy mustard (smooth, not grainy)
2 teaspoons hot curry powder
½ teaspoon onion powder
½ teaspoon salt (optional)
6–8 Spanish olives, sliced

DIRECTIONS
Slice hard-boiled eggs in half lengthwise; remove the yolks and set the whites aside. By hand or in a food processor, mash the yokes to a fine consistency. Add mayonnaise, mustard, curry powder, and onion powder; blend thoroughly until smooth. If necessary, add a little more mayonnaise to get a smooth consistency.

Taste to see if the mixture needs salt. Usually salt is not needed, but that depends on the mustard. Spoon the mixture in a pastry bag* and pipe it into the egg whites. Garnish each egg with an olive slice.

*Instead of a pastry bag, fill a sealable bag. Spoon the mixture into the bag, and twist it to remove air. Cut off a corner, and pipe from that.

VARIATIONS
Smoked Salmon Eggs: Follow directions for curried eggs, omitting mustard, curry powder, salt, and olives. Add ¼ cup finely minced smoked salmon and juice and zest of ½ lemon, and garnish with capers.

Dilled Eggs: Follow directions for curried eggs, omitting mustard, curry powder, and olives. Add 1 tablespoon chopped fresh dill and garnish with dill.

Smoky Bacon Eggs: Follow directions for curried eggs, omitting mustard, curry powder, salt, and olives. Add 2 strips minced turkey bacon (naturally cured) and ¼ teaspoon cayenne pepper (optional).

DR. Z's FAST AND EASY SNACKS

These combinations provide one serving of two or three food groups.

1 hardboiled egg
1 medium apple
CALORIES: 155

1 apple, sliced
2 tablespoons almond butter
CALORIES: 180

¼ cup hummus
1 medium carrot
CALORIES: 135

¼ cup hummus
8 rice crackers
CALORIES: 206

¼ cup blueberries
½ cup strawberries
CALORIES: 80

½–¾ cup broccoli
¼ cup hummus
CALORIES: 115

8 brown-rice crackers
1 serving non-starchy vegetable
1 apple
CALORIES: 176

4–5 brown-rice crackers
¼ cup guacamole *(see recipes)*
CALORIES: 145

4–5 brown-rice crackers
¼ cup Jalapeño-Apple Salsa *(see recipes)*
CALORIES: 100

4–5 brown-rice crackers
¼ cup Mango & Black-Bean Salsa *(see recipes)*
CALORIES: 110

4–5 brown-rice crackers
¼ cup Tomato Relish *(see recipes)*
CALORIES: 110

DR. Z's "JUST WING IT" SALADS

Have you ever wondered how someone can make a mouthwatering meal out of just a few foods and spices, all without measuring or following a recipe? Well, you can too. The following salad recipes are designed to let you create them. If you want more romaine lettuce in the recipe, go for it. If you would rather have more red cabbage than green cabbage, make it your way. You create the recipe you want. You can't mess this up. Just add and subtract ingredients until you get the salad you want.

Look to see what's in your fridge. Use whatever vegetables you have. Mixing different kinds of greens can be tasty; don't be afraid to throw it all together.

When making any of these salads, make enough for leftovers. Before adding the dressing, take what you will eat now, and then store the rest, well covered, in the refrigerator for another meal. Putting dressing over the whole salad will make the leftovers very soggy.

The dressing recipe is perfect for all the salads. Save time by making enough dressing for several salads.

Note: When the recipe calls for legumes, fats, grains, or protein, use them sparingly. For example, if you put a can of butter beans into a big salad, be aware you won't eat the whole can of beans at one meal. The same principle applies to hard-boiled eggs. Eat roughly the right amount of protein, legumes, and fat per serving size.

Vinaigrette Dressing

SERVES 2

CALORIES PER SERVING: 120

INGREDIENTS

2 tablespoons cold-pressed extra-virgin olive oil
1–2 tablespoons cider vinegar (Bragg—see Resources)
1 tablespoon balsamic vinegar
⅛ teaspoon Himalayan or Celtic sea salt
⅛ teaspoon freshly ground black pepper

DIRECTIONS

Combine olive oil and both vinegars; shake to mix well. Season to taste with salt and pepper. This recipe makes ¼ to ⅓ cup of dressing. Adjust the amounts to make more or less.

Use just enough dressing to wet the leaves; they should look shiny but not dripping with oil. This will prevent you from eating too much oil at one meal.

"This Rocks" Salad

CALORIES PER SERVING: 73 PLUS DRESSING

INGREDIENTS

Mixed greens
Romaine lettuce, shredded
Grape tomatoes
Cucumber, sliced or chopped
Carrots, sliced or chopped
Butter beans
Black olives
Fresh green peas
White onion, chopped
Red bell peppers
Hard-boiled egg, if you want protein

Mediterranean Salad

CALORIES PER SERVING: 219 PLUS DRESSING

INGREDIENTS
Romaine lettuce, shredded
White onion, chopped
Mixed olives
Sundried tomato
Artichoke hearts
Butter beans
Red bell pepper

Crunchy Cabbage Salad

CALORIES PER SERVING: 131 PLUS DRESSING

INGREDIENTS
Red and green cabbage, shredded
Carrot, sliced or chopped
Snap peas
Red bell pepper
Cucumber, sliced
Grape tomato
Red onion, chopped

Healthy Heart Salad

CALORIES PER SERVING: 348 PLUS DRESSING

INGREDIENTS
Cauliflower, coarsely chopped
Broccoli, coarsely chopped
Carrot, sliced or chopped
Red onion, chopped
Jicama, chopped (if you want)
Dried cranberries (sweetened with juice, not sugar)
Sunflower seeds

Pantry Salad

This one varies depending on my mood and what I have in the refrigerator, but I will give you one recipe to use as a starting point. Get creative with your own taste buds!

When putting this one together, use more lettuce and spinach. Also use one medium to large carrot. If you don't like a strong onion taste, use a very small onion. Be creative here and use what you have.

CALORIES PER SERVING: 110 PLUS DRESSING

INGREDIENTS
Spring mix lettuce
Spinach
Mushroom
Asparagus
Green beans
Carrot
Celery
Tomato
Broccoli
Red/yellow pepper
Onion, red or white
Red cabbage

Kale Salad

CALORIES PER SERVING: 331 PLUS DRESSING

INGREDIENTS
Kale
Spinach
Apple, chopped
Walnut
Carrot, sliced or chopped
Dried cranberries (sweetened with juice, not sugar)

Egg & Avocado on Toast

SERVES 2

CALORIES PER SERVING: 265

INGREDIENTS
2 slices brown-rice bread (usually found in the frozen-foods
    section of the grocery)
1–2 teaspoons grapeseed oil
2 eggs
¼ ripe avocado, mashed

DIRECTIONS
Toast the brown-rice bread to the consistency you like. Brown-rice bread is not chewy like white Italian bread; don't expect that same texture.

Prepare the eggs the way you like. I like them fried, scrambled,* or boiled and sliced.

Spread mashed avocado over the bread, and add the eggs on top.

*If you usually add milk when scrambling eggs, substitute a non-dairy milk substitute (unsweetened almond or rice milk). I suggest adding nothing but your favorite seasoning. I like Bragg's Organic Sprinkle (see Resources).

EGG & OLIVE SALAD

SERVES 1

CALORIES PER SERVING: 279

INGREDIENTS
2 eggs, hard-boiled
2 tablespoons mayonnaise
¼ teaspoon mustard (Dijon is good, but any mustard will do)
4–6 green olives with pimentos, sliced
~ Freshly ground black pepper

DIRECTIONS
Chop the eggs in an egg slicer (slice lengthwise and crosswise). In a small bowl, mix all ingredients together. Taste and adjust seasoning. Because of the olives, you will probably not need to add salt.

EGGPLANT TAPENADE

This is a versatile recipe. Use as a spread with rice crackers, stuffed into steamed kale leaves, or as a side dish with chicken or fish.

SERVES 6

CALORIES PER SERVING: 110

INGREDIENTS

1 large eggplant
1 large red onion
1 large red bell pepper
3 tablespoons grapeseed oil
~ Sea salt
~ Freshly ground black pepper
1 teaspoon Italian seasoning
2 tablespoons balsamic vinegar
6 cloves garlic (optional)
10 kalamata olives, pitted (or Italian green olives)
1–2 tablespoons olive brine (optional)
~ Pinch of dried oregano
~ Red-pepper flakes (optional)

DIRECTIONS

Preheat oven to 400°.

Dice eggplant, onion, and bell pepper into dime-sized pieces. In a large bowl, combine vegetables with remaining ingredients. Spread mixture on a cookie sheet (covered with foil for easy cleanup) and bake until vegetables are roasted to a creamy texture; this can take up to one hour. Stir every 20 minutes to be sure roasting is even. For a rustic texture, serve just as it comes out of the oven.

For a smoother texture, blend in a food processor, along with olives, brine, and oregano. This version is often called eggplant caviar.

FANTASTIC SPINACH

A versatile side dish, this is a great addition to almost any meal. For breakfast, top it with a poached egg.

SERVES 4

CALORIES PER SERVING: 115

INGREDIENTS

3 tablespoons grapeseed oil
1 large bag organic baby spinach
6 large cloves garlic, chopped
2 shallots, minced (or 1 tablespoon dried onion chips)
1 lemon, juiced
~ Sea salt
~ Freshly ground black pepper

DIRECTIONS

In a large skillet, heat oil over medium heat; add garlic and shallots. Stir until garlic and shallots are slightly browned, which will produce a nutty fragrance. Lower the heat. Stir in lemon juice, salt, and pepper. Add fresh spinach, and toss to get all the leaves coated and gently cooked. In order to preserve the fresh green color, be sure not to overcook.

FEISTY BREAKFAST MEDLEY

SERVES 2

CALORIES PER SERVING: 217

INGREDIENTS

1–2 teaspoons grapeseed oil
3 egg whites plus 1 whole egg
½ cup diced sweet potato, cooked
¼ cup chopped yellow or white onion
½ cup chopped green leafy vegetables (spinach, or frozen
    leafy greens such as collard greens, mustard greens, and
    kale)
¼ cup chopped white button mushroom
¼ cup chopped grape tomatoes
~ Sea salt
~ Freshly ground pepper
~ Red-pepper flakes (optional)

DIRECTIONS

In a medium skillet, heat grapeseed oil. When the oil is hot,
add the egg whites and whole egg. Once the egg starts to
solidify, add remaining ingredients. Mix well while cooking;
be sure the eggs cook completely. Season with a dash of sea
salt, pepper, and, if you like, red-pepper flakes.

VARIATION

Instead of sweet potato, use ½ cup cooked brown rice. Cook
the rice ahead of time. Mix it with the other ingredients, or
serve the mixture over the rice.

FLOURLESS ALMOND-BUTTER COOKIES

MAKES ABOUT 20 COOKIES

CALORIES PER SERVING (1 COOKIE): 119

INGREDIENTS

¾ cup coconut palm sugar (lower glycemic index than cane
     sugar)
½ teaspoon baking soda
¼ teaspoon salt
1 cup creamy-style almond butter
1 large egg, lightly beaten
¾ cup raw almonds, chopped
¼ cup unsweetened, shredded coconut (optional)

DIRECTIONS

Preheat oven to 350°.

In a large bowl, mix together coconut palm sugar, baking soda, and salt. Add almond butter and beaten egg; stir until well combined. Add chopped almonds and shredded coconut (if desired); stir until evenly distributed.

Spoon about 1 tablespoon of dough. With wet hands, roll the dough into a ball and place on an ungreased baking sheet.* Do the same with the rest of the dough, spacing the cookies about 1½ inches apart.

Bake about 15 minutes until they are slightly puffed and have a cracked look on top. Cool for 5 minutes on the baking sheet; any longer will cause them to overcook. Transfer cookies to a rack to finish cooling.

*In order to prevent the cookies from sticking, line the baking sheet with parchment paper. It will also assure that the cookies brown evenly.

VARIATION

Flourless Peanut-Butter Cookies: Follow directions above for almond-butter cookies, substituting 1 cup creamy-style peanut butter for the almond butter, and ¾ cup chopped roasted salted peanuts for the chopped raw almonds. When baking, space the cookies about one inch apart. These do not spread much as they bake. If you have a problem with peanut allergies, skip this recipe.

FRESH FRUIT AND MINT SALAD

SERVES 6

CALORIES PER SERVING: 105

INGREDIENTS
1 pint blueberries
½ pound strawberries, sliced
½ pint raspberries
3 ripe kiwis, sliced in rounds
1 cup sliced red grapes
½ lime, juiced
4 mint leaves, ribbon-sliced

DIRECTIONS
Wash all fruit and cut as noted above. In a large bowl, mix fruit with lime juice and mint leaves.

GLUTEN-FREE BANANA MUFFINS

MAKES 12 MUFFINS

CALORIES PER MUFFIN: 208 (ADDING OPTIONAL INGREDIENTS WILL
INCREASE CALORIE COUNT)

INGREDIENTS
2 cups almond flour
1 cup coconut flour
1½ teaspoons baking soda
3 large eggs
½ teaspoon vanilla extract
½ teaspoon sea salt
2 tablespoons agave nectar
2 tablespoons coconut oil (plus more for greasing the
    muffin tin)
2 cups smashed ripe bananas

optional:
1 cup fresh or frozen blueberries
1 cup coarsely chopped walnuts
¾ cup dark bittersweet chocolate chips

DIRECTIONS
Preheat oven to 350°.

In a large bowl, mix flours and baking soda. In a separate bowl, whisk together eggs, vanilla, salt, agave nectar, and 2 tablespoons coconut oil. When that is thoroughly mixed, add it to the flour mixture and mix until smooth. Fold in the smashed bananas until evenly mixed.

Add any optional ingredients if you choose, and mix well.

Grease a muffin tin with coconut oil. Fill each cup to the rim; the muffins will not rise very much. Bake for 35 minutes. Insert a knife or toothpick into the center of a few muffins; if it comes out clean, they are done. If not, bake for another 10 minutes and check again.

Cool muffins before removing from the tin.

GRILLED KABOBS—CHICKEN, BEEF, OR LAMB

SERVES 2

CALORIES PER SERVING: 270

INGREDIENTS

Marinade
2 tablespoons grapeseed oil
¼ cup white-wine vinegar
1 tablespoon onion powder
2 teaspoons garlic powder
2 teaspoons steak seasoning
~ Sea salt and black pepper

Kabobs
8 ounces meat (chicken, beef, or lamb)
1 large red onion, cut into pieces
1 pint cherry tomatoes
1 bell pepper, cut into pieces
1 tablespoon grapeseed oil
~ Sea salt and black pepper

DIRECTIONS

In a medium bowl, combine all marinade ingredients. Mix thoroughly.

Cut meat into even-sized cubes. Place in a large sealable bag or a flat-bottomed container. Add marinade, and stir well to be sure all the meat is covered. Marinate 2–3 hours or overnight.

Toss vegetables in grapeseed oil, salt, and pepper.

Assemble kabobs; long skewers are recommended. If using wood skewers, soak them well in water beforehand. Using 4–5 cubes of meat per kabob, alternate meat with the 3 vegetables.

Lightly coat the grill with grapeseed oil to prevent sticking. Heat grill to medium, and cook kabobs 3–4 minutes on each side. Check frequently to avoid overcooking.

GUACAMOLE

SERVES 4-6

CALORIES PER SERVING: 107

INGREDIENTS
2 medium ripe avocados, mashed
1 tablespoon lime juice
1 garlic clove (or 1 teaspoon of minced garlic from a jar)
¾ teaspoon sea salt (or Himalayan salt)
~ Sprinkle dry mustard
1 teaspoon onion powder
1 small tomato, chopped

DIRECTIONS
Blend mashed avocado with lime juice and spices. Add chopped tomatoes and mix. Serve immediately. This makes roughly 1½ cups.

CHUNKY GUACAMOLE

SERVES 4

CALORIES PER SERVING: 95

INGREDIENTS
1 large avocado, pitted and cubed
1 scallion, thinly sliced
1 lime, juiced
1 tablespoon chopped cilantro
¼ red bell pepper, finely diced
1 cup grape tomatoes, quartered
1 teaspoon cumin powder
1 teaspoon garlic powder
1 teaspoon extra-virgin olive oil
1 teaspoon sea salt
~ Hot sauce to taste

DIRECTIONS
Mix all ingredients well and chill before serving.

HEARTY NAVY-BEAN SOUP

SERVES 4

CALORIES PER SERVING: 150

INGREDIENTS

3 15-ounce cans organic navy (or white) beans
1 tablespoon grapeseed oil
4 strips naturally cured turkey bacon, cut in half lengthwise
    and sliced into ½-inch pieces (freeze before to make
    cutting easier)
1 large yellow onion, diced
2 stalks celery, diced
3 medium carrots (cut in half lengthwise, sliced ¼-inch
    thick)
6 cups organic chicken stock
2 teaspoons onion powder
1 teaspoon dried oregano
1 teaspoon black pepper
2–3 teaspoons sea salt
1 bay leaf

DIRECTIONS

Put one can of beans, including the liquid, into a blender; blend until smooth.

In a large stew pot over medium heat, sauté diced turkey bacon in grapeseed oil. Add onion, celery, carrots, and a pinch of salt and pepper. Cook for about 5 minutes until onions soften a bit. Remove mixture from the pot and set aside.

In the same pot, add chicken stock, 2 cans of beans (including liquid) and the blended beans, onion powder, oregano, black pepper, 2 teaspoons salt, and the bay leaf. Cover and bring to a boil; reduce heat to a simmer. Add the bacon-and-vegetable mixture; continue cooking uncovered on low heat. As stock thickens, taste to see if more salt is needed. Simmer until beans are smooth in texture and liquid has thickened to a creamy consistency. This should take about 1 hour.

Remove bay leaf before serving.

HUMMUS

SERVES 6

CALORIES PER ¼-CUP SERVING: 95

INGREDIENTS
2 garlic cloves, chopped
1 15-ounce can chickpeas (garbanzo), salt-free
¼ cup water
2 tablespoons tahini
3 tablespoons lemon juice
½ teaspoon organic tamari soy sauce
½ teaspoon cumin
½ teaspoon ground coriander

DIRECTIONS
In a food processor, puree chopped garlic to a creamy consistency. Add all other ingredients; process until very smooth. Transfer to a bowl and chill for an hour or two. Before serving, garnish with 1 tablespoon of finely chopped parsley, if desired.

JALAPEÑO APPLE SALSA

SERVES 6

CALORIES PER SERVING: 49

INGREDIENTS
3 apples (crispy variety), finely diced
½ red bell pepper, finely diced
~ Juice of one lime
1 tablespoon agave syrup
½ jalapeño pepper, finely diced
½ scallion (green only), thinly sliced
2 tablespoons grated fresh ginger
~ Salt to taste

DIRECTIONS
In a bowl, combine all ingredients; taste to adjust seasoning. Serve chilled with rice crackers or as a sauce for fish or chicken.

KALE & WHITE-BEAN SOUP

A quick soup packed with iron, protein, and nutrient-rich vegetables.
SERVES 8

CALORIES PER SERVING: 105

INGREDIENTS
1 cup sliced carrots (2 medium to large carrots)
2 tablespoons grapeseed oil
1 cup diced yellow onion
4 large garlic cloves (or the equivalent in a jar)
1 32-ounce box organic vegetable broth
1 14.5-ounce can diced tomatoes
1 small can tomato sauce
6–8 cups chopped kale
1 14.5-ounce can cannellini beans, drained

DIRECTIONS
In a small saucepan, add carrots to boiling water; once the carrots are soft, drain and set aside.

In a large soup pot, heat grapeseed oil over medium heat. Add onion and cook for 3–4 minutes. Add garlic and cook another 2–3 minutes. Add vegetable broth, tomatoes, tomato sauce, kale, and cooked carrots. Once the kale is tender, add beans.

Serve immediately.

KITCHEN SINK SOUP

SERVES 6

CALORIES PER SERVING: 90

INGREDIENTS
1 tablespoon sesame oil
1 bunch scallions, sliced from white to green
½ head Savoy cabbage, sliced into ½-inch strips
2 cups fresh string beans, cut into ½-inch pieces
3 large carrots, sliced
1 green pepper, diced
10 medium cremini mushrooms, thinly sliced
2–3 quarts fresh chicken stock
¼ cup teriyaki sauce
½ bunch fresh cilantro, coarsely chopped
⅓ cup fresh ginger, cut large enough to remove
~ Salt and pepper to taste

DIRECTIONS
In a large stock pot, add sesame oil and scallions; sauté for a minute on low to medium heat to soften scallions. Add vegetables and mushrooms; stir together and season with salt and pepper.

As vegetables soften and combine, add chicken stock. Bring the mixture to a boil, then lower to simmer. Add teriyaki sauce, cilantro, and ginger. Continue to simmer for an hour. Taste; add more salt, pepper, or teriyaki sauce as needed.

Before serving, remove the pieces of ginger.

LEMON-FRESH QUINOA with Herbs

SERVES 4

CALORIES PER SERVING: 278

INGREDIENTS
1 cup quinoa
1 lemon, juice and zest
1 green onion, sliced fine (green only)
½ cup chopped parsley
1½ cups sliced grape tomatoes
¼ cup extra-virgin olive oil
~ Sea salt and pepper to taste

DIRECTIONS
Cook quinoa according to the directions on the box. Set aside to cool.

Mix together remaining ingredients; stir into quinoa. Serve chilled or at room temperature.

MANHATTAN CLAM CHOWDER

I usually don't recommend eating pork. However, the amount in this recipe is small and it is organic. Companies like Applegate Farms make bacon without hormones or preservatives. If you would rather not eat pork, use turkey bacon to give the chowder a nice flavor.

This is a family-sized recipe. To make less, simply cut the ingredient amounts in half. Leftovers can be frozen for another meal.

SERVES 8–10

CALORIES PER SERVING: 205

INGREDIENTS

2 tablespoons grapeseed oil
1 cup chopped bacon (or turkey bacon)
1 medium-large onion, chopped
2 cups chopped celery
1 cup chopped green pepper
6 cloves garlic, minced
1 cup bottled clam juice
2 14.5-ounce cans crushed tomatoes
1 cup carrots
2 medium sweet potatoes, cubed
1 bay leaf
1 teaspoon dried thyme
2 tablespoons chopped parsley
~ Salt and black pepper to taste
7–8 cans (6.5 ounces each) chopped or minced clams

DIRECTIONS

In a large soup pot over medium heat, add grapeseed oil and bacon (or turkey bacon); sauté until browned, about 3–4 minutes. Add onion, celery, carrots, pepper, and garlic; sauté for another few minutes. Add all remaining ingredients except clams. Simmer until carrots and sweet potatoes are soft. Add clams and let simmer another 5–10 minutes.

Total cooking time is about 45–50 minutes. Test the consistency of the carrots and sweet potatoes; when they are soft, adjust salt and pepper to taste and serve immediately.

MAGIC COLOR-CHANGING SHRIMP STIR-FRY

SERVES 6

CALORIES PER SERVING: 196

INGREDIENTS

1 tablespoon grapeseed oil
4 cloves garlic, coarsely chopped
1 bunch scallions, sliced
1 tablespoon chopped or grated fresh ginger
¼ red cabbage, shredded
3 stalks celery, thinly sliced
1 cup sliced baby carrots
1 can water chestnuts, drained and sliced
1–2 tablespoons rice vinegar
1–2 tablespoons organic tamari sauce
1½ pounds small shrimp, peeled and deveined
1 tablespoon toasted sesame oil
~ Sea salt

DIRECTIONS

In a large skillet, combine grapeseed oil, garlic scallions, and ginger; sauté for one minute. Add vegetables, vinegar, and tamari sauce; sauté until vegetables are tender.

In separate pan on medium heat, sauté shrimp in toasted sesame oil with a pinch of salt. When the shrimp are just turning pink, remove from pan and set aside.

Add shrimp to the vegetables. Stir as the mixture reheats. The red cabbage will cause the shrimp to turn green.

MANGO & BLACK-BEAN SALSA

A delicious accompaniment to fish or a poached egg.
SERVES 6

CALORIES PER SERVING: 85

INGREDIENTS
1 large semi-ripe mango,* diced
1 8-ounce can black beans, drained and rinsed
1 lime, juiced
¼ red bell pepper, finely diced
1–2 scallions, thinly sliced
1 tablespoon chopped fresh cilantro
~ Dash of extra-virgin olive oil
~ Salt and pepper to taste
~ Hot sauce or diced jalapeño pepper (optional)

DIRECTIONS
Mix all ingredients together. Adjust seasoning with salt, black
pepper, hot sauce, or jalapeño pepper to taste.

Mango is a high-glycemic fruit, so eat sparingly.

MARINATED CHICKEN KABOBS

SERVES 4–6

CALORIES PER SERVING: 535 FOR 4; 357 FOR 6

INGREDIENTS
¼ cup grapeseed oil
½ cup fresh orange juice
~ Juice of 1 lemon
4 garlic cloves, crushed
2 scallions, sliced
1 teaspoon dried oregano
1 teaspoon dried thyme
1 teaspoon sea salt
~ Freshly ground black pepper
4–6 chicken breasts, cut into uniform cubes

DIRECTIONS
In a large flat container or sealable bag, combine first nine ingredients to create a marinade. Add chicken cubes and refrigerate for several hours or overnight. Stir several times to be sure all the meat is covered. If using wooden skewers, allow time to soak them in water before assembling kabobs.

Put chicken cubes on skewers; allow a little space between cubes to ensure proper cooking. Coat the grate with grapeseed oil. Cook kabobs over low to medium heat. Turn over halfway through cooking. They cook quickly; a few minutes on each side should be enough.

MIDDLE-EASTERN BURGER

SERVES 4

CALORIES PER SERVING: 231

INGREDIENTS

1 small yellow onion, finely diced
1 clove garlic, minced
1 tablespoon Bragg Liquid Aminos (see Resources)
1 teaspoon ground cumin
1 teaspoon ground cardamom
1 teaspoon smoked sea salt
~ Freshly ground black pepper
1 pound lean ground beef (grass-fed, organic)

DIRECTIONS

Mix together onion, garlic, and all spices. For a spicier (hotter) flavor, add cayenne pepper or diced jalapeño pepper. Mix well into one pound of ground beef, and form four 4-ounce patties. Sauté or grill until the browned. Be careful not to char the meat, as that makes it very toxic.

Serve with avocado or eggplant caviar.

MUSHROOM & BROCCOLI FRITTATA
SERVES 4–6

CALORIES PER SERVING: 210 FOR 4; 141 FOR 6

INGREDIENTS
1½ cups broccoli, chopped
1 tablespoon grapeseed oil
1 bunch of scallions, sliced from white to green
1 18-ounce package cremini mushrooms, sliced
¼ red bell pepper, minced
1 teaspoon dried oregano
½ teaspoon sea salt
~ Freshly ground black pepper
7 large eggs (preferably organic)
½ teaspoon sea salt
~ Freshly ground black pepper
1 teaspoon onion powder
1 teaspoon grapeseed oil

DIRECTIONS
Steam chopped broccoli just until tender; set aside.

In a 10-inch sauté pan on medium heat, add oil, scallions, mushrooms, red pepper, and a little salt and pepper. Sauté for a few minutes to reduce the moisture. Add steamed broccoli, oregano, and a bit more salt and pepper. Cook for a few minutes until flavors combine; add salt if needed. Remove vegetable mixture from the pan and set aside.

In a medium bowl, add eggs, salt, pepper, and onion powder. Mix well with a fork until all yokes are broken.

Coat the sauté pan with 1 teaspoon grapeseed oil. This will make it easy to remove the frittata when it's cooked. Put a small portion of the egg mixture into the oiled pan; add the vegetable mixture in an even layer. Pour the rest of the egg mixture on top. Using a fork, gently push the vegetables to mix in the egg. Cover with a flat lid, and cook over low heat about 15 minutes. Once the top is set, flip the frittata face down to brown for 5 minutes, uncovered. This will eliminate excess moisture.

POACHED FISH POUCHES

Any type of fish works in this recipe. Suggestions include Dover sole, tilapia, lemon sole, scrod, and red snapper.

SERVES 2

CALORIES PER SERVING: 170

INGREDIENTS

2 fresh (not frozen) fish filets, 4 ounces each
~ Sea salt and black pepper
~ Juice and zest of 1 lemon
1 stalk celery, thinly sliced
1 teaspoon thinly slice ginger root
¼ yellow bell pepper, thinly sliced
1 scallion, thinly sliced
1 teaspoon extra-virgin olive oil
2 pinches of cilantro or parsley

DIRECTIONS

Preheat oven to 350°.

In a bowl, toss the sliced ingredients with the olive oil and a pinch of salt and pepper.

Use a piece of foil about 12x14 inches for each filet. Lay the pieces flat and, if you like, cover each with a slightly smaller piece of parchment paper. Place one filet lengthwise on each piece. Sprinkle with a pinch of salt and pepper, and add lemon juice and zest. Divide the vegetables in half and place on top of fish. Add a pinch of cilantro or parsley on top of each.

To seal the pouches, begin by pulling up the sides (lengthwise) and folding them together at the very top. Fold the ends in to make the pouch airtight. The goal is to create a tent-like pouch with room inside for steam.

Bake in the oven for about 10–15 minutes, depending on the thickness of the fish. Be careful of escaping steam when opening the pouch.

Serve with ½ cup wild rice or quinoa.

POWER OATMEAL

If you have a high level of physical activity, these very nutritious, high-calorie meals may be the way to go. Remember not to eat lots of calories at night. These are meant to be consumed early in the day. They are excellent to eat 60–90 minutes before a workout.

SERVES 1

CALORIES PER SERVING: 400

INGREDIENTS
¾ cup steel-cut oats, cooked
½ scoop protein powder (whey, egg-white, or rice protein)
¼ cup strawberries
¼ cup blueberries
~ Ground cinnamon (optional)

DIRECTIONS
Follow the cooking instructions for steel-cut oats. Add protein powder to the cooked oats; mix thoroughly. Top with berries and a dash of cinnamon.

VARIATIONS
Banana Oatmeal: Follow cooking instructions for steel-cut oats. Mix in ½ cup mashed banana while oatmeal cooks. Stir in 6 chopped walnuts, ¼ teaspoon salt, ½ teaspoon vanilla extract, and 1 teaspoon chia seeds.
CALORIES PER SERVING: 389

Pumpkin Oatmeal: Follow cooking instructions for steel-cut oats. Mix in ¼ cup canned pumpkin (unsweetened) while oatmeal cooks. Stir in 1 teaspoon pumpkin-pie spice (or cinnamon), ¼ teaspoon salt, 1 teaspoon chia seeds, and 1 tablespoon agave syrup.
CALORIES PER SERVING: 509

POWER PASTA

SERVES 4–6

CALORIES PER SERVING: 514 FOR 4; 343 FOR 6

INGREDIENTS

1 large head broccoli, cut into small pieces
1 tablespoon grapeseed oil
6–8 cloves garlic, smashed and chopped
1 bunch scallions, sliced white to green
½ bunch kale, washed and cut up
~ Sea salt and pepper
1 medium zucchini, shredded
2 teaspoons dried basil
1 teaspoon dried oregano
8 ounces cremini mushrooms, sliced
1 tablespoon extra-virgin olive oil
1 pound brown-rice pasta (tri-color fusilli)

DIRECTIONS

In a large saucepan, steam chopped broccoli until tender. Set aside.

In a large pot, set 6 quarts of water and 1 tablespoon of salt to boil. This will be used to cook the pasta after the sauce is made.

In a large skillet, heat grapeseed oil over medium heat; add garlic and scallions, and stir for 1–2 minutes. Add kale, salt to taste, and sprinkle with water; cook until kale is wilted. Add zucchini, basil, and oregano; cook for 2 minutes. Add mushrooms, salt, and pepper; cook for another 2 minutes, stirring for 1 minute. Add the broccoli and olive oil; reduce the heat, and cook until flavors are combined.

Add the pasta to the pot of boiling water. Cook according to the package directions; do not overcook. Scoop pasta from boiling water into the sauce; allow some of the pasta water to mix in. This will make the mixture moist and add thickener. Cook for another minute, and serve immediately.

QUICK LEMON CHICKEN

SERVES 8

CALORIES PER SERVING: 180

INGREDIENTS

2 pounds skinless and boneless chicken thighs (tender and
tastier than white meat)
1 teaspoon sea salt
1 teaspoon pepper
1 tablespoon grapeseed oil
2 large yellow onions, cut in half and thinly sliced
1 bulb fresh garlic, peeled and coarsely chopped
1 tablespoon dried or fresh rosemary
~ Sea salt
~ Freshly ground black pepper
1 large lemon, juice and zest

DIRECTIONS

Sprinkle salt and pepper on both sides of chicken thighs; lay
them flat in a large oven-safe baking dish.

Preheat oven to 350°.

In a medium skillet on medium heat, add grapeseed
oil, sliced onions, and garlic; cook for a few minutes. Add
rosemary, salt and pepper to taste, and lemon juice. Sauté
until softened; pour over chicken.

Bake for about 40 minutes. Midway through the cooking
process, add lemon zest and spoon pan juices over the top a
few times. The onions and garlic will create a smooth texture,
and the zesty taste of lemon will brighten the flavors.

QUINOA TABOULEH

SERVES 4

CALORIES PER SERVING: 318

INGREDIENTS
1 cup uncooked quinoa
1 pint grape tomatoes, sliced
1 small cucumber,* cut into bite-sized pieces
2 cups chopped flat-leaf parsley (stems discarded)
½ cup chopped fresh mint
¾ cup sliced ripe olives

Dressing
¼ cup lemon juice
¼ cup olive oil
1 teaspoon lemon zest
~ Salt and pepper to taste

DIRECTIONS
In a large saucepan, combine quinoa with 2 cups water. Bring to a boil, cover, reduce heat, and simmer until water is absorbed (about 15 minutes). Cover and refrigerate until chilled. This can be done a day ahead of time.

In a large bowl, combine cooked quinoa, tomatoes, cucumber, olives, parsley, and mint; stir well.

In a small bowl, combine lemon juice, olive oil, and lemon zest. Mix well; add salt and pepper to taste. Toss well with the salad to be sure the dressing is evenly distributed.

This can be refrigerated for 1–2 days without losing flavor or texture.

Lebanese or Japanese cucumbers are best; they have tender skins and a crunchy texture. English cucumbers are also good. If using a regular cucumber, remove the seeds.

RED CABBAGE, ONIONS, & ORANGES

SERVES 4–6

CALORIES PER SERVING: 148 FOR 4; 98 FOR 6

INGREDIENTS
1 tablespoon grapeseed oil
1 large red onion, thinly sliced
1 large yellow onion, thinly sliced
~ Sea salt and pepper to taste
1 medium red cabbage, halved and thinly sliced
~ Juice and zest of 1 large orange
1 tablespoon fresh or dried tarragon

DIRECTIONS
In a large skillet over medium heat, add grapeseed oil, onions, salt, and pepper; cook for a few minutes. Add cabbage; salt to taste, and sauté for 10 minutes, stirring often.

Once the cabbage has cooked down a bit, add the orange juice and tarragon. Stir well, lower heat, and cook for 5 minutes. Taste and add more salt and pepper, if needed.

In the last minute of cooking, add orange zest and stir well. This is a good accompaniment for grilled meat. The antioxidant properties in the cabbage will help to offset the effects of char from the grill.

ROASTED BRUSSELS SPROUTS

SERVES 4

CALORIES PER SERVING: 72

INGREDIENTS
4 cups Brussels sprouts, cut in half
2 small shallots, sliced
1 tablespoon grapeseed oil
2 tablespoons fennel powder (grind seed in coffee grinder)
1 teaspoon onion powder
2 teaspoons sea salt
~ Freshly ground black pepper

DIRECTIONS
Preheat oven to 175°.

In a large bowl, stir all ingredients together; be sure all the sprouts are coated with seasoning. On a cookie sheet with sides, lay out sprouts and put them in a 175° oven for about 40 minutes. Toss a few times so the sprouts are caramelized on both sides.

SALMON SALAD

SERVES 2

CALORIES PER SERVING: 186

INGREDIENTS
1 6-ounce can wild salmon (or 6 ounces cold poached or
    grilled fresh salmon)
¼ cup diced celery
2 tablespoons mayonnaise (or Vegenaise®—see Resources)
½ teaspoon chopped dried dill
~ Salt and pepper to taste
1 teaspoon horseradish (optional)

DIRECTIONS
Mix all ingredients together. Serve chilled with sliced cucumber and tomatoes.

SAUTÉED SALMON & GREEN BEANS

This dinner takes only about 20 minutes.
SERVES 2

CALORIES PER SERVING: 287

INGREDIENTS
Salmon
2 wild salmon filets, 4 ounces each
1 tablespoon grapeseed oil
1 teaspoon lemon juice
½ teaspoon chopped dill

Green Beans
½ pound green beans
1 tablespoon grapeseed oil
1 tablespoon lemon juice
~ Sea salt
~ Freshly ground black pepper

DIRECTIONS
Salmon
In a medium skillet over low heat, add grapeseed oil. When the oil is hot, add filets (skin side down), and sauté for about 10 minutes, turning often. When salmon is almost done, sprinkle with lemon juice and dill. Remove from heat and season with salt and pepper to taste.

Green Beans
In a large skillet over medium heat, add the grapeseed oil. When it is hot, add the green beans and sauté for 1–2 minutes, stirring constantly. Do not let the beans burn.

When the beans are hot—and very slightly browned—add the lemon juice and cover the pan. Reduce heat and steam the beans for about 2–3 minutes, depending on how crisp you like them. Check frequently.

When done, sprinkle with salt and pepper to taste, and serve immediately.

SCRAMBLED EGGS & SUNDRIED TOMATOES

Serve with fruit for a complete breakfast.

SERVES 2

CALORIES PER SERVING: 318

INGREDIENTS

2 teaspoons grapeseed oil
4 large or extra-large eggs
5–6 sundried tomatoes in oil, chopped
~ Sea salt and black pepper to taste

DIRECTIONS

This is a quick one. In a skillet over medium heat, add oil. In a mixing bowl, combine eggs and sundried tomatoes; whisk thoroughly. Add to skillet and cook until eggs are done.

Add salt and pepper to taste.

SEAFOOD LETTUCE TACOS

SERVES 5

CALORIES PER SERVING: 275

INGREDIENTS

10 large lettuce leaves (Bibb or romaine hearts)
1 teaspoon coriander powder
½ teaspoon chili powder
1 teaspoon garlic powder
2 teaspoons grapeseed oil
1 teaspoon sea salt
1 lime, juiced (if using fresh tuna; ½ lime if using canned tuna)
1 teaspoon chopped fresh cilantro
1 small onion, very thinly sliced
½ pound wild salmon, cubed*
½ pound wild tuna, cubed*
2 tablespoons grapeseed oil

DIRECTIONS

Wash and dry each leaf very well. Refrigerate until use to keep them crisp. To shorten romaine leaves, cut off some of the white at the bottom.

In a large bowl, combine the first eight ingredients to create the marinade. Add the cubed fish and marinate for 1 hour, stirring often.

In a large skillet on medium heat, add 2 tablespoons grapeseed oil. Once oil is hot, remove fish from marinade and add to skillet. Cook 5–7 minutes.

Fill each lettuce leaf just as you would a taco. Top with hot sauce, salsa (without sugar), red onion, cilantro, lime juice, pico de gallo, pickled jalapeños, or whatever you prefer. Chunky Guacamole (see recipe) is a good accompaniment.

*For a quick and inexpensive alternative to fresh fish, use 2 5-ounce cans of solid white tuna and 2 5-ounce cans of wild salmon. Drain the fish before marinating.

SESAME BROCCOLI

SERVES 6

CALORIES PER SERVING: 123

INGREDIENTS

2 tablespoons toasted sesame oil
½ bunch scallions, sliced
2 cloves garlic, crushed
1 carrot, thinly sliced
½ red bell pepper, diced
~ Sea salt
2 pounds broccoli florets, split
2 tablespoons mirin (Asian wine) or organic tamari soy
    sauce
1 tablespoon toasted sesame seeds

DIRECTIONS

In a large skillet, combine oil, scallions, and garlic; cook for 1 minute. Add carrot, bell pepper, and a little salt. Cook for a few more minutes, then add broccoli. Stir well to be sure all the vegetables are covered with oil. Add mirin, and sauté for 3 minutes. Stir in sesame seeds.

Garnish with chopped scallions.

SPAGHETTI CARBONARA

SERVES 1 (FOR 2 SERVINGS, MULTIPLY RECIPE EXACTLY)

CALORIES PER SERVING: 478

INGREDIENTS

1 teaspoon grapeseed oil
¼ small onion, chopped fine
1 strip turkey bacon, cut into small pieces
3 ounces brown-rice spaghetti
1 egg, lightly beaten
~ Salt and pepper to taste

DIRECTIONS

In a large pot over high heat, set water to boil for spaghetti. Add a dash of salt if you like.

In a small skillet, heat grapeseed oil, onion, and turkey bacon; sauté until done. Remove from pan and set aside.

In a small bowl, beat egg with a fork until yolk and white are blended. Set aside.

When water is rapidly boiling, add spaghetti to the pot. Cook until done to whatever consistency you want. Be careful not to overcook it; al dente is best for this recipe.

When the spaghetti is done, quickly drain it and transfer it to a large bowl. Immediately add the beaten egg, and mix thoroughly so the hot pasta cooks the egg. Fold in the bacon-and-onion mixture; salt and pepper to taste. Serve immediately.

SPANISH STUFFED PEPPERS

This makes an excellent family dinner, and is also good as leftovers.
SERVES 6–8

CALORIES PER SERVING: 326 FOR 6; 245 FOR 8

INGREDIENTS
6–8 large bell peppers (red, green, yellow, orange)
1 pound ground turkey
~ Smoked sea salt
~ Freshly ground black pepper
1 tablespoon grapeseed oil
1 medium red onion, diced
4 cloves garlic, crushed
10 medium baby portabella (or cremini) mushrooms,
   chopped
1 can diced tomatoes (organic)
2 teaspoons oregano
1 pinch of saffron, if desired
1 cup Spanish olives, thinly sliced (if salt sensitive, omit
   olives)
2 tablespoons chopped fresh cilantro
½ cup uncooked brown jasmine rice
½ cup uncooked wild rice
8 ounces tomato puree (organic)

DIRECTIONS
Preheat oven to 350°. Cut tops off peppers and clean out the insides. Set upright in an oven-safe baking dish. Set tops around the peppers to keep upright. Chop 2 pepper tops to add to the meat and rice mixture. Set aside.

In a large deep skillet, brown the turkey; season with smoked salt and pepper. Remove from the pan and set aside.

In the hot pan, add grapeseed oil, onion, and garlic. Cook 2 minutes over medium heat, stirring often. Do not let garlic brown. Add pepper tops, mushrooms, salt, and pepper. After it cooks down a bit, add diced tomatoes with juice, oregano, cilantro, and saffron (if desired). When heated, add turkey and both kinds of uncooked rice; stir well and simmer for a minute or two. Add olives, and mix well.

Stuff the peppers very full. Top each one with tomato puree to add moisture. Cover with foil; bake at 350° for 40 minutes. Uncover and bake 30 minutes more, or until peppers are tender.

SPICED SWEET-POTATO CUBES

Baking sweet potatoes with spices really intensifies the flavor. This is a healthful part of any meal or snack. This recipe makes great leftovers for your next meal.

SERVES 6–8

CALORIES PER SERVING: 123

INGREDIENTS
2 large sweet potatoes, washed and cubed
2 tablespoons cold-pressed extra-virgin olive oil
1 teaspoon cumin
1 teaspoon sea salt
¼ teaspoon paprika
¼ teaspoon cayenne pepper

DIRECTIONS
Preheat oven to 400°.

In a big mixing bowl, combine cubed sweet potato with olive oil; mix thoroughly so the cubes are somewhat wet with oil. Stir in spices so they are evenly spread throughout the mixture.

On a baking sheet, evenly spread spiced potato cubes. Bake until the cubes are soft, roughly 35–45 minutes. Depending on your oven, this may take more or less time. Check regularly until they are the consistency you want.

SPICY GARLIC HUMMUS

Serve as a snack with rice crackers or vegetables—celery, broccoli, zucchini, cauliflower.

SERVES 12

CALORIES PER SERVING: 95 PER ¼ CUP

INGREDIENTS

2 cans organic chickpeas (garbanzos), drained (save some
   liquid from the can)
4 large cloves garlic
4 tablespoons tahini
1 lemon, juiced and zested
½ teaspoon cayenne pepper
1 teaspoon salt
1 tablespoon extra-virgin olive oil

DIRECTIONS

In a food processor, blend all ingredients until smooth. Add liquid from the can of beans, if necessary, to get a smooth consistency.

SPLIT-PEA SOUP

This keeps well, so it is a great leftover.
SERVES 8–10

CALORIES PER SERVING: 265 FOR 8; 213 FOR 10

INGREDIENTS
3 quarts water
1–1¼ pounds dry split peas
1 ham bone
2 medium onions, finely chopped
2 medium carrots, chopped
2 celery stalks, sliced
1 teaspoon sea salt (or Himalayan salt)
½ teaspoon black pepper
2 small sweet potatoes, diced

DIRECTIONS
In a large soup pot, add all ingredients except sweet potatoes. Bring mixture to a boil; immediately lower heat and simmer for 2 hours. Once the peas fall apart and the carrots are soft, add diced sweet potatoes. Serve once all vegetables are soft.

STRING BEANS & TOMATOES

SERVES 6

CALORIES PER SERVING: 73

INGREDIENTS
2 pounds green beans
~ Sea salt
1 tablespoon grapeseed oil
1 bunch scallions, sliced
~ Freshly ground black pepper
2 cups grape tomatoes, sliced in half
1 teaspoon chopped fresh mint*
1 teaspoon chopped fresh tarragon*

DIRECTIONS
Prepare green beans by snapping off the stem ends and cutting in half crosswise. Put the beans in a large skillet and add water to halfway cover the beans. Season with sea salt. Bring to a boil; remove from heat, cover, and steam for 5 minutes or until tender. Strain, remove from skillet, and set aside.

In the same skillet on medium heat, add grapeseed oil, scallions, a little salt and pepper, grape tomatoes, and tarragon. Cook for a minute; add green beans, fresh mint, and salt and pepper to taste. Cook until tomatoes break down to a creamy consistency.

For a more Italian flavor, use fresh basil instead of mint and tarragon.

SUMMER FRUIT SALAD

SERVES 2

CALORIES PER SERVING: 87

INGREDIENTS
1 cup sliced strawberries
1 cup blueberries
1 peach, sliced and cut in pieces
¼ cup orange juice
5–6 leaves fresh mint, chopped

DIRECTIONS
Combine all ingredients. Set aside for ½ hour to allow flavors to marinate. Drain excess orange juice,* and serve at room temperature. If making this ahead, refrigerate, covered, until ½ hour before serving. The fruits are more flavorful if served at room temperature.

*Drinking the excess orange juice will increase the calorie count. Pure fruit juice is high in sugar.

SUMMER POACHED SALMON

SERVES 4 • CALORIES PER SERVING: 359

Dressing

INGREDIENTS

1 small cucumber, finely diced
1 tablespoon minced fresh dill
½ cup mayonnaise (or Vegenaise®—see Resources)
~ Sea salt
~ Freshly ground black pepper
1 lemon, quartered to sprinkle on fish or as a garnish

DIRECTIONS

Prepare the dressing first, so the flavors can combine. Peel the cucumber and remove seeds; mince the rest. Lightly salt the minced cucumber and set in a strainer to drain. Press with a paper towel to remove water.

In a medium bowl, combine dill, mayonnaise, salt and pepper to taste, and a squeeze of lemon. Set aside to serve at room temperature.

Poached Salmon

INGREDIENTS

3–5 celery stalks
~ Wild salmon, one large filet or 4 steaks
1–2 teaspoons onion powder
~ Sea salt
~ Lemon pepper (or freshly ground black pepper)
1 lemon, sliced
1 bunch fresh dill (leave intact for easy removal)

DIRECTIONS

In a large skillet with a lid, place fish on celery stalks to raise it off the pan. Sprinkle with onion powder, salt, and pepper. Top with lemon slices and whole sprigs of dill. Add water to reach the bottom edge of the fish; *do not submerge fish.* Gently boil for about 15 minutes. When the thickest part of the fish is still a bit darker, turn off heat, cover, and let sit for another 5 minutes.

Remove dill and top with dressing.

SUMMER SALAD

SERVES 4

CALORIES PER SERVING: 370

INGREDIENTS

1 heart of romaine
2 cups mesclun salad
1 carrot, shredded
1 cup snap peas, sliced
½ cup grape tomatoes, cut in half
½ cup black olives, sliced
½ cup yellow or red bell pepper, cut bite-sized
½ bunch flat-leaf parsley, coarsely chopped
3–4 sprigs dill, coarsely chopped
4 basil leaves, chiffonade (rolled and thinly sliced)
¼ cup slivered or sliced almonds
¼ cup pumpkin seeds

Easy Balsamic Dressing
3 tablespoons extra-virgin olive oil
1–1½ tablespoons balsamic vinegar
½ teaspoon garlic powder
½ teaspoon Italian seasoning
¼ teaspoon sea salt
~ Freshly ground black pepper

DIRECTIONS

In a small bowl, whisk together all dressing ingredients. In a large bowl, combine all salad ingredients. Add dressing and toss well to make sure dressing is thoroughly distributed.

SUPER-MOIST TURKEY MEATBALLS

MAKES 45 MEATBALLS

CALORIES PER SERVING: 280 FOR 5 MEATBALLS

INGREDIENTS
¾ cup cooked brown rice
1 cup shredded zucchini
¼ cup chopped fresh parsley
1 tablespoon powdered fennel or seeds
1 teaspoon sea salt
½ teaspoon freshly ground black pepper
2 eggs, lightly beaten
1 tablespoon minced dried onion
2 pounds ground turkey

DIRECTIONS
Preheat oven to 400°.

Place shredded zucchini in a strainer and sprinkle with salt; this will draw out excess water. After about half an hour, press out remaining water through the strainer.

In a food processor, combine rice, zucchini, parsley, fennel, salt, and pepper; pulse until minced to a fine consistency. Blend in eggs and dried onion. Add ground turkey and mix thoroughly.

Roll mixture into 1-inch balls; the consistency will be soft and somewhat mushy. They will not hold a nice round shape, but they taste great. Bake on a cookie sheet for 20 minutes, then broil on high heat until meatballs are browned.

Serve with tomato sauce, or alongside sweet potatoes and vegetables. These also make a good snack. These meatballs keep very well in the freezer; be sure to wrap carefully in sealed freezer bags. To defrost, move them to the refrigerator overnight; place them in a sealable bag in a bowl of cold water for about half an hour, or use the defrost setting in a microwave. Once defrosted, reheat in the oven or in a skillet with tomato sauce.

SWEET MUSHROOM SALAD

SERVES 4

CALORIES PER SERVING: 60

INGREDIENTS

½ lime, juiced
½ scallion, thinly sliced, light green to dark green
1 teaspoon coriander seeds
1 teaspoon cardamom seeds
1 teaspoon agave nectar
1 tablespoon extra-virgin olive oil
~ Sea salt to taste
~ Freshly ground black pepper to taste
16 ounces firm cremini mushrooms, very thinly sliced

DIRECTIONS

Combine the first 8 ingredients; shake well to blend. Pour over mushrooms, and toss well. Marinate in the refrigerator, stirring often. It is best when marinated for at least a half hour, but can be eaten immediately if time is limited.

TACO-LESS TACO SALAD

SERVES 4–6 • CALORIES PER SERVING: 292

INGREDIENTS

1 pound grass-fed ground beef or bison, or organic ground turkey

2 heads romaine lettuce, chopped

2 hearty handfuls spring-mix lettuces, chopped

1 large carrot, shredded

¼ medium white onion, diced

½ red bell pepper, diced

½–¾ medium-large cucumber, diced

¾ cup chopped grape tomatoes, cut in half

½–¾ package of Daiya non-dairy cheese, mozzarella-style shreds

10 large black olives, chopped

1 cup unsweetened mild or moderate salsa

~ Organic, sprouted-grain chips (not tacos)

Taco Spice

2 teaspoons ground cumin

1 teaspoon Himalayan sea salt

1 teaspoon ground black pepper

1 teaspoon paprika

¼ teaspoon onion powder

¼ teaspoon garlic powder

¼ teaspoon crushed red-pepper flakes

¼ teaspoon dried oregano

1 tablespoon chili powder

DIRECTIONS

In a bowl, mix all the spices and set aside. In a large skillet, fry ground meat of choice (beef, bison, or turkey) until cooked through. While still warm, add spice mixture a little at a time; taste and add spice until you like it. Sprinkle the non-dairy cheese over the meat so it melts.

In a large mixing bowl, combine lettuces, bell pepper, carrot, and other vegetables. Put the spiced meat on top, and add organic sprouted chips.

TANGY SALSA & EGGS

SERVES 1

CALORIES PER SERVING: 337

INGREDIENTS
½ cup cooked brown rice
½ cup unsweetened salsa
½ teaspoons grapeseed oil
2 eggs

DIRECTIONS
In a bowl, mix the brown rice and salsa; set aside.
    In a small skillet, fry or scramble the eggs in grapeseed oil.
Add eggs to the rice and salsa mixture.

THAI CURRIED TILAPIA (or chicken)

SERVES 4

CALORIES PER SERVING: 188 FOR FISH; 230 FOR CHICKEN
(ADD 85 FOR RICE)

INGREDIENTS

2 tablespoons coconut oil (1 for garlic and onions and 1 for
    vegetables)
1 tablespoon grated fresh ginger
2 cloves garlic, crushed
½ bunch scallions, thinly sliced
1 medium red onion, halved and thinly sliced
1 tablespoon green curry paste (or red if you
    prefer milder spice)
1 teaspoon sea salt
½ green bell pepper, thinly sliced
½ red bell pepper, thinly sliced
2 carrots, julienned (cut like shoe strings)
1 can water chestnuts, drained and sliced
1 can light coconut milk
4 tilapia filets, 4 ounces each (or 4 chicken breasts,
3 ounces each)
1 tablespoon fresh cilantro, chopped (optional)

DIRECTIONS

In a large sauté pan on low to medium heat, add 1 tablespoon
coconut oil, ginger, garlic, scallions, and onion. Cook for 2
minutes, stirring constantly. Add curry paste and cook for
another 2 minutes. Add 1 more tablespoon coconut oil, salt,
and remaining vegetables. Cook for 4 minutes. Add the
coconut milk and simmer for a few minutes. Add salt, if
needed. Add the tilapia (or chicken) and cover. Cook for 5
minutes; remove cover and cook 5 more minutes. Sprinkle
with fresh cilantro and serve with ½ cup wild rice.

If using chicken, slice it into strips and add to the pan before
the vegetables. Cook for a few minutes, stirring occasionally;
then add the vegetables and follow the rest of the directions.

TOMATO RELISH

Use as an appetizer or snack with rice crackers, or as a sauce over chicken or fish.

SERVES 5

CALORIES PER SERVING: 55 FOR ¼ CUP

INGREDIENTS

2 tablespoons extra-virgin olive oil
1 15-ounce can organic diced tomatoes, drained
1 large red onion, halved and sliced
½ red bell pepper, finely diced
8 large leaves fresh basil, slivered
1 teaspoon dried oregano
~ Sea salt
~ Freshly ground black pepper

DIRECTIONS

In a large skillet over medium heat, add olive oil and sauté onions, oregano, salt, and pepper for 2 minutes. Add bell pepper and cook for another 10 minutes. Lower the heat, add tomatoes, and cook until flavors are combined and onions are tender. Stir in fresh basil, and cook just a bit more.

TOMATO SOUP

SERVES 8–10

CALORIES PER SERVING: 90 FOR 8; 70 FOR 10

INGREDIENTS
3 quarts water
1 soup bone from a grass-fed cow
2 16-ounce cans organic tomato sauce
1 12-ounce can tomato paste
2 teaspoons sea salt (or Himalayan salt)
½ teaspoon black pepper
2 cubes organic beef bouillon (or the equivalent in powder)
4 carrots, chopped
4 celery stalks, chopped

DIRECTIONS
In a large soup pot, add the water, soup bone, and tomato sauce. Once the water boils, turn heat down to simmer. To thicken the soup, add tomato paste a little at a time until you get the consistency you want. Add salt, pepper, and bouillon cubes. Simmer for one hour. Add carrots and celery. Simmer another hour, or until the carrots and celery are soft.

TUNA SALAD

SERVES 2

CALORIES PER SERVING: 232

INGREDIENTS
1 can tuna (American Tuna brand is low in mercury)
1 Fuji apple, chopped
¼ cup dried cranberries (sweetened with juice, not sugar)
2 tablespoons mayonnaise (or Vegenaise®—see Resources)
½ teaspoon mustard, or to taste
~ Freshly ground black pepper

DIRECTIONS
In a medium bowl, mix together tuna, chopped apple, and dried cranberries. Combine mayonnaise and mustard; mix into salad. Season with pepper to taste.

TURKEY & VEGETABLE ONE-DISH SUPPER

SERVES 5

CALORIES PER SERVING: 332

INGREDIENTS
3 tablespoons grapeseed oil
1 medium onion, chopped
3 cloves garlic, peeled and minced (use more or less to taste)
8 ounces mushrooms, rinsed and chopped
¼ cup chicken stock
1 pound ground turkey (dark meat has more flavor)
1 teaspoon celery seed
1 teaspoon dried basil (or fresh in season)
1 28-ounce can diced tomatoes in juice
1 medium to large zucchini, sliced and cut into pieces
1 large bell pepper
1 8-ounce can black olives, drained and sliced
1 teaspoon umeboshi plum vinegar* (optional)

Available in most specialty groceries, this is prevalent in Japanese food. It brightens flavors with a mild citrus-salty note.

DIRECTIONS
In a large skillet over medium heat, put 2 tablespoons grapeseed oil and chopped onion; sauté until soft (about 2–3 minutes). Add garlic and cook until onions are translucent (2–3 more minutes); do not let garlic burn. Add mushrooms and chicken stock; cook for about 5 minutes. Add salt and pepper to taste. Remove mixture from the pan and set aside.

In the same skillet over medium heat, add 1 tablespoon grapeseed oil and ground turkey. As it cooks, break up the meat so it cooks uniformly. Add celery seed and dried basil; sauté until meat is cooked through, about 5 minutes. Reduce heat, and return the vegetable mixture to the pan. Add tomatoes and juice. Mix well; adjust seasoning with salt and pepper. While the mixture simmers, add zucchini; it will cook as the liquid reduces. Add ripe olives and umeboshi vinegar (if desired); simmer for about 10 more minutes to reduce the liquid. Just before serving, adjust the seasoning one more time.

TURKEY BOLOGNESE

SERVES 5–6

CALORIES PER SERVING: 392

INGREDIENTS

2–3 teaspoons grapeseed oil
1 pound ground turkey, dark or light meat
1 25-ounce jar organic tomato sauce
1 12-ounce bag brown-rice pasta (penne or fusilli)

DIRECTIONS

Fill a soup pot with water and bring to a boil. If you like, add a teaspoon of grapeseed oil to help prevent the pasta from sticking together.

In a skillet, heat 2 teaspoons grapeseed oil over medium heat. Add ground turkey, stirring it until evenly cooked. Stir in tomato sauce and continue cooking until the sauce is hot. Reduce heat to keep the sauce warm while the pasta cooks.

Once the water is boiling, add the pasta. When the water appears milky, check the pasta to see if it is cooked to the consistency you like, al dente, or softer.

Drain the pasta and place in a large serving bowl; stir in the turkey sauce, and serve immediately. Alternatively, divide the pasta into individual serving bowls, and top with the sauce.

TURKEY CONFETTI BOWL (or Beef)

SERVES 6

CALORIES PER SERVING: 285

INGREDIENTS
2 cups shredded zucchini
3 cups cooked wild rice
1 large red onion
1 red bell pepper
1 ear fresh corn (or 1 cup frozen shoe-peg corn)
1 pound ground turkey (or 1 pound grass-fed ground beef)
~ Sea salt
~ Pepper
1 tablespoon grapeseed oil
5 large basil leaves, chopped
1 jalapeño pepper, chopped (optional)

DIRECTIONS
Toss shredded zucchini with salt and set aside in a strainer to drain. This should be done ahead of time to allow time for the moisture to drain.

Cook wild rice according to package directions.

Cut onion and bell pepper into chunks. In a food processor, chop them into smaller pieces and set aside. Process them separately to get uniform pieces. This can also be done by hand.

Cut corn kernels off the cob; set aside.

In large deep skillet, brown the meat with 1 teaspoon salt and pepper. Remove from pan and set aside.

In the same skillet over medium heat, add grapeseed oil, onion, and a pinch of salt. Cook until onion is soft, then add bell pepper, zucchini, and jalapeño pepper (if desired). Cook for about 10 minutes. Add cooked rice, meat, corn, and basil; cook for 5 minutes until flavors combine. Adjust salt and pepper to taste.

TUSCAN BEAN DIP

Serve with rice crackers or gluten-free toasted bread cut into triangles. Both will add to the calories, so check labels carefully. Avoid rice crackers containing sugar or potato starch.

SERVES 6

CALORIES PER ¼ CUP SERVING: 78

INGREDIENTS

1 tablespoon extra-virgin olive oil
8 large cloves garlic, smashed and coarsely chopped
2 teaspoons crushed dried oregano
~ Sea salt to taste
1 15-ounce can small white beans (reserve ½ cup can liquid)
~ Freshly ground pepper
~ Red-pepper flakes (optional)

DIRECTIONS

In a saucepan on low heat, combine olive oil, garlic, oregano, and salt. Cook very slowly until garlic is soft and golden in color. Add beans and ½ cup liquid from the can. (Water or vegetable broth can be substituted for the can liquid.) Let beans cook until liquid thickens. Add salt and pepper to taste, and red-pepper flakes, if desired.

To increase the recipe, just add a second can of beans.

TUSCAN CABBAGE, KALE, & BEANS

This is a delicious vegetarian main dish, or as a side dish with beef, lamb, or poultry. It is also good with a poached egg for breakfast.
SERVES 6

CALORIES PER SERVING: 334

INGREDIENTS
2 tablespoons olive oil
1 bulb garlic, peeled and coarsely chopped
1 tablespoon sea salt
1 teaspoon freshly ground black pepper
2 teaspoons dried oregano
2 8-ounce cans organic white northern beans (or 16 ounces of
    home-cooked navy beans and their cooking juice)
1 medium yellow onion, quartered and sliced
1 head Savoy cabbage, quartered, sliced ¼-inch
½ bunch kale, stems removed and finely chopped
1 teaspoon red-pepper flakes (optional)

DIRECTIONS
In a small saucepan, place 1 tablespoon grapeseed oil and all the garlic; cook until tender. Add a pinch of salt, pepper, the oregano, and both cans of beans, including the liquid. Cook for 10 minutes uncovered on low heat; cover and cook for 10 more minutes until beans are tender. Add more salt for flavor if needed. This mixture will supply most of the flavor in the recipe.

In a large sauté pan on medium heat, heat 1 tablespoon grapeseed oil. Add onion, salt, and pepper; cook until tender. Add all the cabbage and kale; sprinkle lightly with water to create steam. Stir, cover, and cook for 1 minute; repeat those steps until the cabbage is tender but not too soft. Add the bean mixture; stir well and cover. Turn off heat and set aside to allow the flavors to combine. Season with red-pepper flakes, if desired.

VEGETABLE STIR-FRY

SERVES 2–3

CALORIES PER SERVING: 167 FOR 2; 111 FOR 3

INGREDIENTS

1 tablespoon grapeseed oil
1 large onion, diced
3 cloves garlic, finely chopped
1 teaspoon fresh chopped ginger
1 carrot, slices
2 stalks celery, cut into ¼-inch slices
1 large head broccoli, cut into small pieces
1 can sliced water chestnuts
1 cup snap peas, whole or cut
1 teaspoon sesame oil
1 tablespoon organic tamari soy sauce

DIRECTIONS

In a large skillet over medium heat, add grapeseed oil, onion, garlic, and ginger; cook for one minute, stirring constantly to avoid burning. Add all vegetables and a pinch of salt and pepper; cook for 2 minutes. Add tamari soy sauce and cook for another 2 minutes. Add sesame oil and salt and pepper to taste; stir well and transfer to a platter to avoid overcooking.

WALDORF SALAD

SERVES 6

CALORIES PER SERVING: 183

INGREDIENTS

2 red-skinned apples (Pink Lady or Gala), cut into bite-sized pieces

2 cups red grapes, halved

4 stalks fresh celery, sliced ¼-inch thick

½ small red onion, sliced thin

½ cup coarsely chopped walnuts

~ Juice of 1 lemon

¼ cup mayonnaise (or Vegenaise®—see Resources)

DIRECTIONS

In a large bowl, combine all ingredients except mayonnaise. Add mayonnaise and mix well.

VARIATIONS

Make this salad a main dish by adding steamed or grilled chicken. Vary the flavor by adding fresh tarragon or mint.

ZUCCHINI PANCAKES

SERVING: 6–8 TWO-INCH PANCAKES

CALORIES PER SERVING: 174

INGREDIENTS

3 cups shredded zucchini
1 cup cooked brown rice
¼ cup shredded dried coconut
½ bunch fresh scallions, sliced white to light green
⅓ cup raisins
1 teaspoon grated fresh ginger
1 tablespoon curry powder
2 teaspoons sea salt (or to taste)
2 eggs, lightly whisked
3 tablespoons brown-rice flour
1 can water chestnuts, drained and coarsely chopped
1 tablespoon grapeseed oil

DIRECTIONS

Sprinkle shredded zucchini with salt and place in a strainer to drain excess water. After about half an hour, press out remaining water through the strainer.

Put first eight ingredients into a food processor and blend to a grainy consistency.

In a large bowl, whisk eggs with brown-rice flour. Add the zucchini mixture and water chestnuts; mix well.

In a nonstick skillet over medium heat, add the grapeseed oil. Once oil is heated, make one pancake to test the consistency. If it does not hold together, stir another teaspoon of brown-rice flour into the batter, and taste to see if more salt is needed. Cook remaining pancakes in batches. Five cups of batter makes about 30–35 pancakes (approximately 6 pancakes per cup).

If well sealed, the batter can be refrigerated for a few days before cooking. It also freezes well, if divided into several batches.

Product Recommendations and Resources

Throughout this book, you will occasionally see recommendations for certain products that I find beneficial and superior in some way. Here I have described those products and provided information on where to locate them.

Vegenaise® — This is a vegan mayonnaise substitute made without artificial ingredients. It has a very pleasant, clean flavor. Whether or not you are a vegan, you may like this product. Some think it tastes more like homemade mayonnaise than commercial brands. It is available in most natural-foods stores and some supermarkets, as well as online at www.followyourheart.com.

Daiya Non-Dairy Cheese — This is the only dairy-free cheese I have found that does not contain traces of casein, a milk protein. It can be found in natural-foods stores and online at www.daiyafoods.com.

Bragg Liquid Aminos — A certified non-GMO (not genetically modified), gluten-free liquid protein concentrate derived from soybeans, this is an excellent and healthful seasoning for almost any type of food. It can be ordered online at www.bragg.com/products.

Nuts — Organic, raw nuts which have been soaked and gently dried are much easier to digest and have greater health benefits than nuts usually found in stores. They are available online at www.livingnutz.com.

Wild Seafood — I recommend that you eat only wild seafood, available at many natural-foods stores and some supermarkets. The website www.vitalchoice.com has a complete selection, as well as other organic foods.

Grass-Fed Meats — Like seafood, the type of meat you eat is very important for your health. I recommend only grass-fed, naturally raised meat, available at www.uswellnessmeats.com, as well as natural-foods stores and some supermarkets.

Nutritional Supplements — For further information on advanced, science-based nutritional supplements, please contact me at www.drzembroski.com.

References

Decide

Almanac of Chronic Disease, 2008 Edition.

Paul M. Ridker, MD, Eleanor Danielson, MIA, Francisco A. H. Fonseca, MD, Jacques Genest, MD, Antonio M. Gotto Jr., MD, John J. P. Kastelein, MD, Wolfgang Koenig, MD, Peter Libby, MD, Alberto J. Lorenzatti, MD, Jean G. MacFadyen, BA, Borge G. Nordestgaard, MD, James Shepherd, MD, James T. Willerson, MD, and Robert J. Glynn, ScD, for the JUPITER Study Group. Rosuvastatin to Prevent Vascular Events in Men and Women with Elevated C-Reactive Protein. *The New England Journal of Medicine*, 2008; 359; 21.

World Cancer Research Fund/American Institute for Cancer Research. Food, Nutrition, Physical Activity, and the Prevention of Cancer: A Global Perspective. Washington, DC: AICR, 2007.

Preetha Anand, Ajaikumar B. Kunnumakara, Chitra Sundaram, Kuzhuvelil B. Harikumar, Sheeja T. Tharakan, Oiki S. Lai, Bokyung Sung, and Bharat B. Aggarwal. Cancer Is a Preventable Disease That Requires Major Lifestyle Changes. *Pharmaceutical Research*, 2008; 25; 9.

Anne C. Chiang, MD, PhD, and Joan Massagué, PhD, Molecular Basis of Metastasis. *New England Journal of Medicine*, 2008;259:2814–23.

Edward Giovannucci. Insulin, Insulin-Like Growth Factors and Colon Cancer: A Review of the Evidence. *The Journal of Nutrition*, 131:3109S-3120S, 2001.

Edward Giovannucci. Insulin and colon cancer. *Cancer Causes and Control*, 1995 March;6(2):164-79.

Lee S. Gross, Li Li, Earl S. Ford, and Simin Liu. Increased Consumption of Refined Carbohydrates and the Epidemic of Type 2 Diabetes in the United States: An Ecological Assessment. *The American Journal of Clinical Nutrition*, 2004; 79:774–779.

Eric Steen, Benjamin M. Terry, Enrique J. Rivera, Jennifer L. Cannon, Thomas R. Neely, Rose Tavares, X. Julia Xu, Jack R. Wands, and Suzanne M. de la Monte. Impaired Insulin and Insulin-Like Growth Factor Expression and Signaling Mechanisms in Alzheimer's Disease—Is This Type 3 Diabetes? *Journal of Alzheimer's Disease*, 2005; 7:63–80.

Indulge

A. Janet Tomiyama, PhD, Traci Mann, PhD, Danielle Vinas, BA, Jeffrey M. Hunger, BA, Jill DeJager, MPH, RD, and Shelley E. Taylor, PhD. Low Calorie Dieting Increases Cortisol. *Psychosomatic Medicine*, 2010; 72:000–000.

Martin O. Weickert and Andreas F. H. Pfeiffer. Metabolic Effects of Dietary Fiber Consumption and Prevention of Diabetes. *The Journal of Nutrition*, 2008; 138:439–442.

Alexandra M. Johnstone, Graham W. Horgan, Sandra D. Murison, David M. Bremner, and Gerald E. Lobley. Effects of a High-Protein Ketogenic Diet on Hunger, Appetite, and Weight Loss in Obese Men Feeding Ad Libitum. *The American Journal of Clinical Nutrition*, 2008; 87:44–55.

Peter S. Ungar, Frederick E. Grine, and Mark F. Teaford. A Review of the Evidence and a New Model of Adaptive Versatility. *Annual Review of Anthropology*, 2006; 35:209–228.

Katharine Milton. The Critical Role Played by Animal Source Foods in Human (Homo) Evolution. *The Journal of Nutrition*, 2003; 133:3886S–3892S.

Susan L. Teitelbaum, Marilie D. Gammon, Julie A. Britton, Alfred I. Neugut, Bruce Levin, and Steven D. Stellman. Reported Residential Pesticide Use and Breast Cancer Risk on Long Island, New York. *American Journal of Epidemiology,* 2007;165;643-651.

Roberto Ferro, Arvin Parvathaneni, Sachin Patel, Pramil Cheriyath. Pesticides and Breast Cancer. *Advances in Breast Cancer Research,* 2012, 1, 30-35.

Felix Grün and Bruce Blumberg. Environmental Obesogens: Organotins and Endocrine Disruption via Nuclear Receptor Singaling. *Endocrinology,* 2006 147:s50-s55.

Environmental Health Perspectives, Vol. 120;2:February 2012.

M. P. Richards. A Brief Review of the Archaeological Evidence for Palaeolithic and Neolithic Subsistence. *European Journal of Clinical Nutrition,* 2002, 56.

C. Daniel Smith, MD, Sharon B. Herkes, PhD, Kevin E. Behrns, MD, Virgil F. Fairbanks, MD, Keith A. Kely, MD, and Michael G. Sar, MD. Gastric Acid Secretion and Vitamin B12 Absorption After Vertical Roux-en-Y Gastric Bypass for Morbid Obesity. *Annals of Surgery,* 218; 1:91–96.

E. Ginter. Chronic Vitamin C Deficiency Increases the Risk of Cardiovascular Diseases. *Bratislava Medical Journal,* 2007; 108; 9:417–421.

Marco N. Diaz, MD, Balz Frei, PhD, Joseph A. Vita, MD, and John F. Keaney, Jr., MD, Antioxidants and Atherosclerotic Heart Disease. *New England Journal of Medicine,* August 1997, 408.

Dianne E. Coder. Worldwide Increasing Incidences of Cutaneous Malignant Melanoma, *Journal of Skin Cancer,* 2011, Article ID 858425.

Wei Zhu, Donglian Cai, Ying Wang, Ning Lin, Qingqing Hu, Yang Qi, Shuangshuang Ma, and Sidath Amarasekara.

Calcium Plus Vitamin D3 Supplementation Facilitated Fat Loss in Overweight and Obese College Students with Very-Low Calcium Consumption: A Randomized Controlled Trial. *Nutrition Journal*, 2013, 12:8.

Loren Cordain, PhD. Cereal Grains: Humanity's Double-Edged Sword. *The World Review of Nutrition and Dietetics,*1999; 84:19–73.

Kristin K. Deeb, Donald L. Trump, and Candace Johnson. Vitamin D Signaling Pathways in Cancer: Potential for Anticancer Therapeutics. *Nature Reviews,* September 2007, 7:684.

Cedric F. Garland, DrPH, FACE, Edward D. Gorham, MPH, PhD, Sharif B. Mohr, MPH, and Frank C. Garland, PhD, Vitamin D for Cancer Prevention: Global Perspective. *Annals of Epidemiology,* July 2009; 19; 7:468–483.

Sanjeev Kumar Syal, MD, Aditya Kapoor, DM, Eesh Bhatia, MD, DNB, Archana Sinha, MSc, Sudeep Kumar, DM, Satyendra Tewari, DM, Naveen Garg, DM, Pravin K. Goel, DM. Vitamin D Deficiency, Coronary Artery Disease, and Endothelial Dysfunction: Observations From a Coronary Angiographic Study in Indian Patients. *Journal of Invasive Cardiology*, 2012; 24; 8:385–389.

Klevay LM. Heart Failure improvement from a supplement containing copper. *European Heart Journal*, 2006 Jan;27(1):117.

Center for Disease Control and Prevention: Iron Deficiency. www.cdc.gov.

R. S. Rivlin. Magnesium Deficiency and Alcohol Intake: Mechanisms, Clinical Significance and Possible Relation to Cancer Development (a Review). *Journal of the American College of Nutrition*, 1994; 13; 5:416–423.

Ka He, Liancheng Zhao, Martha L. Daviglus, Alan R. Dyer, Linda Van Horn, Daniel Garside, Liguang Zhu, Dongshuang

Guo, Yangfeng Wu, Beifan Zhou, and Jeremiah Stamler for the INTERMAP Cooperative Research Group. Association of Monosodium Glutamate Intake with Overweight in Chinese Adults: The INTERMAP Study. *Obesity*, 2008; 16:1875–1880.

De-Yi Liu, Boon-Shih Sie, Ming-Li Liu, Franca Agresta, and H. W. Gordon Baker. Relationship Between Seminal Plasma Zinc Concentration and Spermatozoa-Zona Pellucida Binding and the ZP-Induced Acrosome Reaction in Subfertile Men. *Asian Journal of Andrology*, 2009; 11:499–507.

Tiina H. Rissanen, Sari Voutilainen, Kristiina Nyyssönen, Riitta Salonen, George A. Kaplan, and Jukka T. Salonen. Serum Lycopene Concentrations and Carotid Atherosclerosis: The Kuopio Ischaemic Heart Disease Risk Factor Study. *The American Journal of Clinical Nutrition*, 2003; 77:133–138.

Franco O. Ranelletti, Nicola Maggiano, Fabrio G. Serra, Riccardo Ricci, Luigi M. Larocca, Paola Lanza, Giovanni Scambia, Andrea Fattorossi, Arnaldo Capelli, and Mauro Piantelli. Quercetin Inhibits p21-RAS Expression in Human Colon Cancer Cell Lines and in Primary Colorectal Tumors. *International Journal of Cancer*, 2000; 85; 3:438–445.

Yu-quan Wei, Xia Zhao, Yoshitaka Kariya, Hideki Fukata, Keisuke Teshigawara, and Atsushi Uchida. Induction of Apoptosis by Quercetin: Involvement of Heat Shock Protein. *Cancer Research*, 1994; 54:4952–4957.

Taylor C. Wallace. Anthocyanins in Cardiovascular Disease. *Advances in Nutrition*, 2011; 2:1–7.

Maria R. Cesarone, MD, Andrea Di Renzo, Silvia Errichi, MD, Frank Schönlau, PhD, James L. Wilmer, PhD, and Julian Blumenfeld, MD. Improvement in Circulation and in Cardiovascular Risk Factors with a Proprietary Isotonic Bioflavonoid Formula OPC-3®. *Angiology*, 2008; 59; 408.

The Relationship of Dietary Carotenoid and Vitamin A, E, and C Intake With Age-Related Macular Degeneration in a Case-Control Study. *Archives of Ophthalmology,* 2007;125(9):1225-1232

Carolyn M. Cover, S. Jean Hsieh, Erin J. Cram, Chibo Hong, Jacques E. Riby, Leonard F. Bjeldanes, and Gary L. Firestone. Indol-3-Carbinol and Tamoxifen Cooperate to Arrest the Cell Cycle of MCF-7 Human Breast Cancer Cells. *Cancer Research,* March 15, 1999; 59:1244–1251.

Carolyn M. Cover, S. Jean Hsieh, Susan H. Tran, Gunnell Hallden, Gloria S. Kim, Leonard F. Bjeldanes, and Gary L. Firestone. Indole-3-carbinol Inhibits the Expression of Cyclin-Dependent Kinase-6 and Induces a G1 Cell Cycle Arrest of Human Breast Cancer Cells Independent of Estrogen Receptor Signaling. *The Journal of Biological Chemistry,* 1998; 273; 7:3838–3847.

Baiba J. Grube, Elizabeth T. Eng, Yeh-Chih Kao, Annette Kwon, and Shiuan Chen. White Button Mushroom Phytochemicals Inhibit Atomatase Activity and Breast Cancer Cell Proliferation. *The Journal of Nutrition,* 2001; 131:3288–3293.

Christopher M. Lockwood, Jordan R. Moon, Sarah E. Tobkin, Ashley A. Walter, Abbie E. Smith, Vincent J. Dalbo, Joel T. Cramer, and Jeffrey R. Stout. Minimal Nutrition Intervention with High-Protein/Low-Carbohydrate and Low-Fat, Nutrient-Dense Food Supplement Improves Body Composition and Exercise Benefits in Overweight Adults: A Randomized Controlled Trial. *Nutrition & Metabolism,* 2008; 5:11.

Kathleen M. Fairfield and Robert H. Fletcher. Vitamins for Chronic Disease Prevention in Adults: Scientific Review. *The Journal of the American Medical Association,* 2002; 287; 23.

Loren Cordain, PhD. Cereal Grains: Humanity's Double-Edged Sword. *The World Review of Nutrition and Dietetics,* 1999; 84:19–73.

J. L. Outwater, A. Nicholson, and N. Barnard. Dairy Products and Breast Cancer: The Estrogen, and bGH Hypothesis. *Medical Hypothesis*, 1997; 48:453–461.

Jolieke C. van der Pols, Chris Bain, David Gunnell, George Davey Smith, Clare Frobisher, and Richard M. Martin. Childhood Dairy Intake and Adult Cancer Risk: 65-Y Follow-Up of the Boyd Orr Cohort. *The American Journal of Clinical Nutrition*, 2007; 86:1722–1729.

Norie Kurahashi, Manami Inoue, Motoki Iwasaki, Shizuka Sasazuki, and Shoichiro Tsugane for the Japan Public Health Center–Based Prospective Study Group. Dairy Product, Saturated Fatty Acid, and Calcium Intake and Prostate Cancer in a Prospective Cohort of Japanese Men. *Cancer Epidemiology, Biomarkers & Prevention*, 2008; 17:930–937.

Amy Joy Lanou, PhD; Susan E. Berkow, PhD, CN; and Neal D. Barnard, MD. Calcium, Dairy Products, and Bone Health in Children and Young Adults: A Reevaluation of the Evidence. *Pediatrics*, 2005; 115; 3.

Diane Feskanich, ScD, Walter C. Wilet, MD, DrPH, Meir J. Stampfer, MD, DrPH, and Graham A. Colditz, MD, DrPH. Milk, Dietary Calcium, and Bone Fractures in Women: A 12-Year Prospective Study. *American Journal of Public Health*, 1997;87:992-997.

Fazlul H. Sarkar and Yiwei Li. Using Chemopreventive Agents to Enhance the Efficacy of Cancer Therapy. *Cancer Research*, 2006;66(7):3347-50.

Marco N. Diaz, MD, Balz Frei, PhD, Joseph A. Vita, MD, and John F. Keaney, Jr., MD. Antioxidants and Atherosclerotic Heart Disease. *The New England Journal of Medicine*, August 7, 1997, 408.

Jia-Yi Dong, Pengcheng Xun, MD, PhD, Ka He, MD, Li-Qiang Qin, MD, PhD. Magnesium Intake and Risk of Type 2 Diabetes. *Diabetes Care*, 34:2116-2122, 2011.

R Jayawardena, P Ranasinghe, P Galappatthy, RLDK Malkanthi, GR Constantine, and P Katulanda. Effects of zinc supplementation on diabetes mellitus: a systematic review and meta-analysis. *Diabetology & Metabolic Syndrome*, 2012, 4:13.

Hamid R. Farshchi, Moira A. Taylor, and Ian A. MacDonald. Deleterious Effects of Omitting Breakfast on Insulin Sensitivity and Fasting Lipid Profiles in Healthy Lean Women. *The American Journal of Clinical Nutrition*, 2005; 81:388–396.

S. Bilz, R. Ninnis, and U. Keller. Effects of Hypoosmolality on Whole-Body Lipolysis in Man. *Metabolism*, 1999; 48; 4:472–476. PubMed.

D. Häussinger, E. Roth, F. Lang, and W. Gerok. Cellular Hydration State: An Important Determinant of Protein Catabolism in Health and Disease. *Lancet*, 1993; 22:341. PubMed.

U. Keller, G. Szinnai, S. Bilz, and K. Berneis. Effects of Changes in Hydration on Protein, Glucose and Lipid Metabolism in Man: Impact on Health. *European Journal of Clinical Nutrition*, 2003; 57, Suppl. 2, S69–S74.

Michael R. Irwin, Carmen Carrillo, and Richard Olmstead. Sleep Loss Activates Cellular Markers of Inflammation: Sex differences. *Brain, Behavior, and Immunity*, 2010 January;24(1): 54-57.

Michael R Irwin, MD; Minge Wang, MSN; Capella O. Campomayor, MS; Alicia Collado-Hidalgo, PhD; Steve Cole, PhD. Sleep Deprivation and Activation of Morning Levels of Cellular and Genomic Markers of Inflammation. *Archives of Internal Medicine*, 2006;166;1756-1762.

Enjoy

Hamid R. Farshchi, Moira A. Taylor, and Ian A. MacDonald. Deleterious Effects of Omitting Breakfast on Insulin Sensitivity and Fasting Lipid Profiles in Healthy Lean Women. *The American Journal of Clinical Nutrition,* 2005; 81:388–396.

P. Björntorp. Do Stress Reactions Cause Abdominal Obesity and Comorbidities? *Obesity Reviews,* 2001; 2:73–86.

Elissa S. Epel, PhD, Bruce McEwen, PhD, Teresa Seeman, PhD, Karen Matthews, PhD, Grace Castellazzo, RN, BSN, Kelly D. Brownell, PhD, Jennifer Bell, BA, and Jeannette R. Ickovics, PhD. Stress and Body Shape: Stress-Induced Cortisol Secretion Is Consistently Greater Among Women with Central Fat. *Psychosomatic Medicine,* 2000; 62:623–632.

Transform

B. K. Pedersen and B. Saltin. Evidence for Prescribing Exercise as Therapy in Chronic Disease. *Scandinavian Journal of Medicine & Science in Sports,* 2006; 16; Suppl. 1:3–63.

Yukihito Higashi, Shota Sasaki, Satoshi Kurisu, Atsunori Yoshimizu, Nobuo Sasaki, Hideo Matsuura, Goro Kajiyama, and Tetsuya Oshima. Regular Aerobic Exercise Augments Endothelium-Dependent Vascular Relaxation in Normotensive as Well as Hypertensive Subjects: Role of Endothelium-Derived Nitric Oxide. *Circulation,* 1999; 100:1194–1202.

Ingo Helmich, Alexandra Latini, Andre Sigwalt, Mauro Giovanni Carta, Sergio Machado, Bruna Velasques, Pedro Ribeiro, and Henning Budde. Neurobiological Alterations Induced by Exercise and Their Impact on Depressive Disorders. *Clinical Practice & Epidemiology in Mental Health,* 2010; 6:115–125.

Pierpaolo De Feo, Chiara Di Loreto, Anna Ranchelli, Cristina Fatone, Giovanni Gambelunghe, Paola Lucidi, and Fausto Santeusanio. Exercise and Diabetes. *Acta Biomed,* 2006; 77; Suppl. 1:14–17.

Jason L. Talanian, Stuart D. R. Galloway, George J. F. Heigenhauser, Arend Bonen, and Lawrence L. Spriet. Two Weeks of High-Intensity Aerobic Interval Training Increases the Capacity for Fat Oxidation During Exercise in Women. *Journal of Applied Physiology*, 2007; 102:1439–1447.

Robert H. Coker, PhD, Rick H. Williams, MS, Patrick M. Kortebein, MD, Dennis H. Sullivan, MD, and William J. Evans, PhD. Influence of Exercise Intensity on Abdominal Fat and Adiponectin in Elderly Adults. *Metabolic Syndrome and Related Disorders*, 2009; 7:363–368.

Anne McTiernan, Shelley S. Tworoger, Cornelia M. Ulrich, et al. Effect of Exercise on Serum Estrogens in Postmenopausal Women: A 12-Month Randomized Clinical Trial. *Cancer Research*, 2004; 64:2923–2928.

Lis Adamsen, Morten Quist, Christina Andersen,Tom Møller, Jørn Herrstedt, Dorte Kronborg, Marie T Baadsgaard, Kirsten Vistisen, MD, Julie Midtgaard, Birgitte Christiansen, Maria Stage, Morten T. Kronborg, Mikael Rørth. Effect of a multimodal high intensity exercise intervention in cancer patients undergoing chemotherapy: randomized controlled trial, *British Medical Journal*, 2009;339:b3410.

Ingrid C. De Backer, Eric Van Breda, Art Vreugdenhil, Marten R. Nijziel, Arnold D. Kester and Goof Schep. High-intensity strength training improves quality of life in cancer survivors. *Acta Oncologica*, 2007; 46:1143-1151.

Bente Klarlund Pedersen and Laurie Hoffman-Goetz. Exercise and the Immune System: Regulation, Integration, and Adaptation. *Physiological Reviews*, Vol. 80, No. 3, July 2000.

Gabriella Barclay, Tim Shiraev, Clinical Benefits of High-Intensity Interval Training. *Australian Family Physician*, Vol. 41, No. 12, December 2012.

Arnt Erik Tjønna, MSc, Sang Jun Lee, PhD, Øivind Rognmo, MSc, Tomas O. Stølen, MSc, Anja Bye, MSc, Per Magnus

Haram, PhD, Jan Pål Loennechen, PhD, Qusai Y. Al-Share, MSc, Eirik Skogvoll, PhD, Stig A. Slørdahl, PhD, Ole J. Kemi, PhD, Sonia K. Najjar, PhD, Ulrik Wisløff, PhD, Aerobic Interval Training Versus Continuous Moderate Exercise as a Treatment for Metabolic Syndrome. *Circulation*, 2008; 118:346–354.

Angelo Tremblay, Jean-Aime Simoneau, and Claude Bouchard. Impact of Exercise Intensity on Body Fatness and Skeletal Muscle Metabolism. *Metabolism*, 1994; 43:814–818.

M. Yoshioka, E. Doucet, S. St-Pierre, N. Alméras, D. Richard, A. Labrie, J. P. Després, C. Bouchard, and A. Tremblay. Impact of High-Intensity Exercise on Energy Expenditure, Lipid Oxidation and Body Fatness. *International Journal of Obesity*, 2001; 25:332–339.

Mark D. Schuenke, Richard P. Mikat, and Jeffrey M. McBride. Effect of an Acute Period of Resistance Exercise on Excess Post-Exercise Oxygen Consumption. *European Journal of Applied Physiology*, 2002; 86:411–417.

J. A. Kanaley, J. Y. Weltman, J. D. Veldhuis, A. D. Rogol, M. L. Hartman, and A. Weltman. Human Growth Hormone Response to Repeated Bouts of Aerobic Exercise. *Journal of Applied Physiology*, 1997; 83:1756–1761.

Fabio S. Lira, Luiz C. Carnevali Jr., Nelo E. Zanchi, Ronaldo V. T. Santos, Jean-Marc Lavoie, and Marília Seelaender. Exercise Intensity Modulation of Hepatic Lipid Metabolism. *Journal of Nutrition and Metabolism*, doi:10.1155/2012/809576.

Michael J. Ormsbee, John P. Thyfault, Emily A. Johnson, Raymond M. Kraus, Myung Dong Choi, and Robert C. Hickner. Fat metabolism and acute resistance exercise in trained men. *Journal of Applied Physiology*, 2007; 102:1767–1772.

About the Author

Dr. Robert Zembroski is a Chiropractic Physician, Board-Certified Chiropractic Neurologist, Clinical Nutritionist, specialist in functional medicine, author and public speaker. Twenty years in private practice has helped Dr. Zembroski become an expert in health topics, including heart disease, diabetes, obesity, cancer, and hormone-related issues. He specializes in treating neurological and musculoskeletal dysfunctions, as well as acute and chronic pain syndromes. He also educates and counsels his patients on therapeutic lifestyle changes to help them manage and overcome their health issues. Currently, Dr. Zembroski is the director of The Darien Center for Functional Medicine, in Darien, Connecticut.

For more information:
www.drzembroski.com
www.darienfm.com